ONE THOUSAND MUSTACHES

ONE THOUSAND MUSTACHES

A CULTURAL HISTORY OF THE MO

ALLAN PETERKIN

Arsenal Pulp Press | Vancouver

ARSENAL PULP PRESS
Suite 101, 211 East Georgia St.
Vancouver, BC V6A 1Z6
Canada
arsenalpulp.com

The publisher gratefully acknowledges the support of the Canada Council for the Arts and the British Columbia Arts Council for its publishing program, and the Government of Canada (through the Canada Book Fund) and the Government of British Columbia (through the Book Publishing Tax Credit Program) for its publishing activities.

Efforts have been made to locate copyright holders of source material wherever possible. The publishers welcomes hearing from any copyright holders of material used in this book who have not been contacted.

Book design by Gerilee McBride
Mustache illustrations (pp. 126–135) by Jaye Lyonns
Cardboard mustaches by Angela Caravan
Editing by Susan Safyan
Author photograph by Robert Thomas
Printed and bound in Canada

Library and Archives Canada Cataloguing in Publication

Peterkin, Allan D.
    One thousand mustaches : a cultural history of the mo / Allan Peterkin.

Includes bibliographical references and index.
Issued also in electronic format.
ISBN 978-1-55152-474-0

    1. Mustaches—Social aspects—History. 2. Mustaches—History.
I. Title.

GT2318.P48 2012   391.5   C2012-904417-2

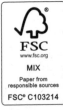

FSC
www.fsc.org
MIX
Paper from
responsible sources
FSC® C103214

CONTENTS

INTRODUCTION

When my first book on the subject of facial hair, *One Thousand Beards*, was published in 2001, I somewhat tentatively predicted the return of the mustache. In the years that followed, what we saw instead (at least initially) was further "growth" of the beard in cheeky variations, like the play-off beard, the strike beard, the lay-off beard, the break-up beard, and the mountain-man beard. The long-neglected mo, on the other hand, could be spotted on an occasional fashion runway, on the face of a feckless sitcom character, or on your Uncle Fitz, where it had been comfortably situated for years. The brave fellow who grew one spontaneously in his natural habitat had to cope with layer upon layer of historical projections—was he a fop (i.e., hopelessly effete), a foreigner (a term favored by clean-shaven men of pallor), or a fiend (twirling the tips with evil on his mind)? He would also be reminded that barbarians wore them as they sacked Rome (which permanently set the standard for the ferocious military mustache thereafter); that tired old colonials wore them as the Empire collapsed; that Charlie Chaplin boasted one as the bumbling Tramp; and that members of the seminal '70s disco group Village People wore different variations as they encouraged young men to explore their local YMCA.

The mustache, then, an iconic symbol of adventure, virility, and fierce independence, had been "tarnished" or at least become complicated. To wear a stache was to face an endless stream of unwelcome questions and comments. But little by little, the status of the stache improved, thanks to pioneers and proponents like the Handlebar Club, the American Mustache Institute, the Glorius [*sic*] Mustache Challenge, the World

Beard and Mustache Championships, and charitable initiatives like Movember (an Aussie-originated fundraiser for prostate cancer research that has spread worldwide like wildfire in recent years). The ubiquitous beard-mania that reached new heights with the goatee in the mid-'90s more than paved the way for the PoMo mo. Men realized that their faces were blank canvases and that they were suddenly free to express themselves at home and at work in ways their fathers and grandfathers (who were often corporate nine-to-five slaves) could not. Facial hair was meant to be playful, masculine, sexy, and ironic. You did it with a wink of an eye (and a twirl of your waxed tips) and could actually revel in the ways your furry face got misread, ridiculed, or fetishized by those around you.

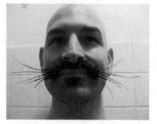

Keith J. Haubrich's cat whiskers (self-portrait) won 1st place in the Freestyle Mustache category at the World Beard & Moustache Championships 2007 in Brighton, UK.

The mustache has thus become a spectacular, embodied performance of masculinity in all its post-millennial complexity and ambiguity. To wear a stache is to wear your personality on your sleeve (or in this case, your face).

So, stache-wearers, it's time to take back the mo from evil dictators and porn stars and to embrace this elegant choice of facial hair full on. It's time to remind others that it's not all about the beard. More mo's for everyone!

Moustache is the British spelling, while mustache is American. Canadians (ever-obliging) use both spellings.

WHY MEN WILL ALWAYS GROW MUSTACHES

Over time, the rationale for stache-growing has morphed as the popularity of the mustache has waxed and waned. These are the most common reasons men have tended to sport lip fur and still do:

- because a mustache is masculine and virile (and studies prove it!)
- it's less upkeep than a full beard
- it's a form of playful rebellion or provocation (against parents, the workplace, and general clean-shavenness)
- because your favorite historical figures have worn one (Gandhi, Martin Luther King Jr.)
- it's a professional norm (e.g., military, police, firefighter, lion-tamer)
- it's a symbol of national pride (Poles, Spaniards)
- it's an emblem of war
- your favorite movie or sports star wears one
- your president / prime minister / king had one (William Taft / Robert Borden / Charlemagne)
- it acts as an air filter and keeps your upper lip warm
- it's always a conversation starter

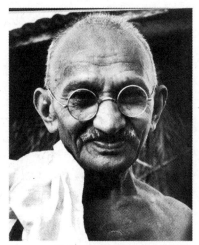

Mahatma Gandhi, in the 1940s.

- it keeps others guessing about your sexuality (gay, bi, swinger)
- it's the last frontier of facial hair (everything else has been done since goatees hit in the '90s)
- it statistically increases your chance of getting married (and has done so for centuries, based on recent research)
- it's a form of adolescent pride (peach fuzz and the first wisps of facial hair)
- it's fun to wax, twirl, and play with it
- it makes you part of a stache-brotherhood (like the American Mustache Institute)
- it's a personal trademark
- it's a family tradition (your dad had one, and his dad afore him)
- because your partner is pro-mo
- it helps to mark a transition (divorce, new job, wanting to look older or younger)
- it balances your facial features (like a big nose)
- it changes your public face (why did Alex Trebek of *Jeopardy!* shave his?)
- it's great for charity (Movember, Mustaches for Kids)
- it shows support for your teams during playoffs
- it's a useful disguise

Until the 1940s, a man had plural "mustaches." Now he has but one "mustache."

THE MO WE KNOW

The average human male has about five million follicles—about three times as many as gibbons and gorillas, but still less than the chimpanzee.

Average human hair grows at a rate of 0.014 inches per day, or about five to six inches per year.

Average length and growth rate per day:

Hairs on the scalp 0.35 mm

Eyebrows: 0.15 mm

Mustaches: 0.4 mm

Armpit hairs: 0.3 mm

Pubic hairs: 0.2 mm

Most men have about 25,000 whiskers.

A mustache is capable of absorbing twenty percent of its own weight in liquid.

There are between 10,000 and 20,000 hairs on a man's entire face.

Ninety percent of men shave once a day.

Shaving uses up five months of a man's life if he starts at the age of fourteen.

A man will shave approximately 20,000 times over a lifetime.

Sixty percent of men use disposable razors; twenty percent use electric.

Razors and blades are a $1.1 billion industry.

An eighty-year-old man has likely spent 2,965 hours of his life shaving.

Mustache development is determined by genetics and hormones so there's little you can do to affect the qualities of your facial hair or the patterns of its growth.

Facial hair (barring eyebrows) is least dense on the lower cheek, most dense on the upper lip (the stache wins again!).

Facial hair protrudes at a thirty-five to fifty-five degree angle.

Mustache hair grows at a faster rate in the spring and summer than in autumn and winter.

A 2008 poll showed that 61.2 percent of respondents found the mustache to be gentlemanly and sophisticated, while 38.9 percent believed it was worn only by fools and fiends.

The average mustachioed man touches his mo 760 times every twenty-four hours.

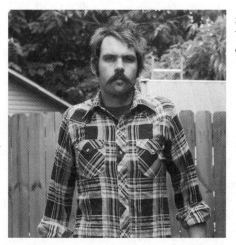

Self-portrait of Jonathan Youngblood, illustrating the concept "hipster," 2009.

A "crustache" is the wispy growth on the upper lip of a teen, hipster, or trailer-park resident.

MUSTACHE SYNONYMS OVER THE AGES

There are numerous slang terms for the mustache. Most reflect its resemblance to a variety of animals, its tendency to retain food and drink, or its association with sexual activity.

Bristle batons	Lip lettuce
Bro-mo	Lip shadow
Bro-stache	Lip spinach
Cookie duster	Lip sweater
Crumb catcher	Lip waterfall
Crustache	Lower brow
Double hamster	Manometer
Face-fittings	Mamma's little helper
Face-lace	Mo
Face fungus	Mobile tea strainer
Face shelf	Mouser
Face spanner	Moustachio
Facial furniture	Mouth-stache
Fanny duster	Mouthbrow
Flavor-saver	Moz
Grass grin	Mr Tickles
Handlebars	Muzzy
Lady tickler	Nose bug
Lip doily	Nose neighbor
Lip fur	Pushbroom
Lip fuzz	Snot catcher

Soup strainer	Trash stash
Stache	Upper lipholstery
Stash	Waxed affair
Strip-teaser	Whiskers
Tache	Wing
Tash	Womb broom
Tea strainer	

A mustache "twiddler" or "twirler" is an epithet for a villain.

THE MO IN ANCIENT HISTORY

In the beginning, there was a mustache. Cave-boys became cave-teens who sprouted mustaches on their way to developing beards. Adam himself would have had a mustache before he had a beard. We know this because, in the natural onset of human puberty, facial hair grows first at the corners of the upper lip. Bit by bit, new hair fills in the gap above the lip, completing a full-on mustache. Under the influence of testosterone, the lowly beard is an inevitability thereafter, as hair grows on the upper part of the cheeks and below the lower lip. It soon fills in the lower chin, sides of the face, and neck to create the bushy look we most associate with Neanderthals or contemporary mountain men. Not only does the mustache come first in human history, but it also represents an elegant balance between young and old, the smooth female face and the overly furry male face. Its horizontal line marks up and down, heaven and hell, who's in and who's out.

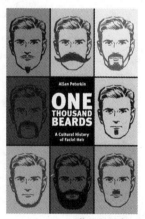

Allan Peterkin,
One Thousand Beards, 2001.

Compared to the many tomes that have been written about the beard throughout history, including my own book *One Thousand Beards*, there are relatively few serious books on the mustache as a specific, stand-alone entity. Often paintings, sculptures, and artifacts from a particular era are the only available record of the stache's popularity (or very existence) during that period.

Details on the evolution of lip whiskers as a style are indeed scant. For most of history (and as is still often the case), the beard and mustache came as a single package governed by religious, political, class, and social conventions. Of course, all boys grew what modern hipster critics now call the "crustache," i.e., wispy strands upon an otherwise smooth face. The pre-hirsute teens were usually told to be patient and wait for the real thing—the full beard. Somewhere along the line, however, someone had the bright idea to shave the lower face and leave the hairy lip celebrated and untouched. As early as 2650 BCE, Egyptian artifacts revealed men sporting a pencil-thin line of hair on their upper lips, perhaps in admiration of the cat—they were worshippers of feline forms. But by 1800 BCE, they again became clean shaven; legend has it that one "Pharaoh Teqikencola" banned them outright. (No reason for this mo-radication has been documented.) A fastidious lot the Egyptians were; removing all body hair was essential, as it was seen as base and beastly. Nonetheless, both kings and queens would at times enjoy wearing lavish fake beards made of gold and silver called *postiches*, which were strapped behind the ears like a Halloween mask. Queen Hatshepsut

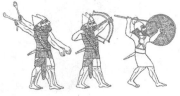

Assyrian soldiers.

(circa 1480 BCE) herself wore a dazzling pleated variant that left no doubt as to who was boss. Her slaves were clean shaven, so as to be readily identified; this was one of the first times in history that we know that the absence or presence of facial hair was an immediate signifier of social status, a practice that would recur over time.

In the seventh century BCE, the Assyrians wore beards and wigs dyed with henna or pitch and often powdered with gold dust. Upper-crust beards had tiny curls, arranged in three hanging tiers. Soldiers, by contrast, were instructed to keep their chins trimmed in due deference, but this did not include mustaches, so theirs may be the first military mo's.

The Persians favored short pointed beards dyed red and woven with gold threads. They fought one of the first beard wars when the Tatars tried to get them to wear a religious beard style that they didn't like. The Tatars also despised the Persians' mustaches. (Although the Persians fussed over their long, luxurious mustaches, they were infrequent bathers and seldom washed their hair.) However, the stache was a Persian trademark, and they can be considered the first real heroes in mustachioed history.

Most famous Greeks—from their philosophers to their lightning-throwing gods—had excellent beards. (In general, hair had tremendous significance for the ancient Greeks, particularly after death, when it was cut, torn out, or burned by grieving relatives.) Upper-class Greek boys did not cut their facial hair until their staches and beards started to grow, at which point they were cut and sacrificed to Apollo. Greek men competed fiendishly over the coif and elegance of their facial hair; whoever had the most skilled trim-servant (barber) was victor. It is ironic that the word "mustache" comes from the Doric Greek *mystax*, meaning upper lip. The Greeks may have named them, but they refused to wear them without accompanying beards!

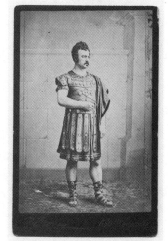

American actor Edwin Forrest, in costume as the character Spartacus, ca. 1872.

The Spartans, however, underscored the masculinity of the mustache in their laws; those convicted of cowardice had half of their mustaches removed to evoke instant public stigma and shame. (Clearly, this was a symbolic form of castration.)

----•◦•----

Greek historian Herodotus presumed that the shaven and mustachioed Scythians were smitten with a strange disease that made them resemble women because of spiritual misbehavior.

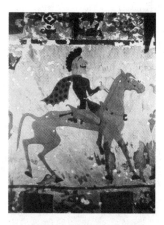

A popular image shows a Pazyryk horseman (ca. 300 BCE), who proudly displays his tribal stache.

While Greece was beginning to enjoy its Golden Age in the sixth century BCE, in China a most scholarly mustache was being sported by Confucius, born in 551 BCE, and by most of the early great Chinese philosophers that followed him. Confucius allegedly said, "A man without a mustache is a man without a soul." Depictions of Lao Tzu (also sixth century, BCE), the founder of philosophical Taoism, show him wearing a mustache (and a long beard), too. But in popular Chinese operas of a later era, villains and men of the lower classes were portrayed with mustaches. Rich but dubious playboy characters were often identifiable by their pencil-thin versions, their mo's a symbol of wealth, sophistication, and dodgy intentions.

While the Greeks disdained the mustache in the absence of the beard, the Romans must have cursed its very existence as they fought off the barbaric and magnificently mustachioed Goths, Gauls, and Franks while they sequentially plundered Rome. Youthful Franks were not allowed to trim the hair on their faces or heads at all until they made their first kill, showing they were war-ready. In no small measure, we have these pre-French barbarian tribes to thank for bringing us *le moustache français* that has defined them ever since. The Gaulish aristocrats wore staches while commoners wore beards. To get an idea of what the Gauls, in what later became France, looked like, check out a famous statue called *The Dying Gaul* (at the Capitoline Museum in Rome), which shows a muscular young man with a fine mustache bravely resisting his demise.

The ancient Britons also wore droopy mustaches, often dyed green or blue as an act of defiance against Caesar. (Contrary to popular opinion, these marauders and pillagers were not called barbarians because they had *barbes*. The word originated from a term that signified "un-Greek" and when uttered aloud sounded like someone massacring the Greek language.) Julius Caesar commented on their use of colored powder in their facial hair. The ancient Gauls also associated long tresses with great honor. When Julius Caesar subdued them and made them shave their heads in submission, this was yet another historical example of symbolic castration involving hair.

The name Algernon comes from the Old French *aux gernons*, meaning "to have mustaches."

Early Romans, meanwhile, were hairy but not mustachioed. They repeatedly insisted that their beard styles were "less feminine than the Greeks." When a slew of Greek-Sicilian barbers arrived in Rome in 297 BCE, shaving became all the rage until Emperor Hadrian (117–138 CE) grew a beard to hide his facial scars and warts and, of course, everyone followed suit with copycat beards. Young Romans were quite peacockish, letting their teen fuzz-beards grow until they reached the age of maturity, when they shaved them off. Like their Greek forebears, they consecrated their beards to the gods.

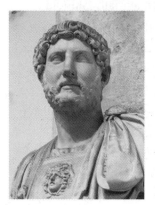

Emperor Hadrian
Musei Capitolini, Rome.

The Emperor Nero even placed his shaven whiskers in a stunning gold box encrusted with pearls. Facial hair took on added significance when Romans in mourning let their beards grow wild and unruly after the death of a loved one.

Roman slaves had no choice about growing or shaving the hair on their own faces. They were subjected to shaving when beards were chic; when beards went out of fashion, they were expected to grow them. This made slaves easy to spot if they tried to run away. And while the upper classes had their own in-house shave slaves, barbershops ready to serve the average fellow sprouted everywhere. Barbershops were a hub for gossip, socializing, and getting the latest gladiator scores.

The Romans may have inadvertently helped the mustache along because they were the first to use warm water, an oily form of shaving cream, and a straight razor to shave. The great Roman general Scipio Africanus (236–183 BCE) is thought to have been the first Roman to shave daily—up to three times a day, in fact. The next three Roman emperors thereafter—Hadrian, Antoninus Pius, and Marcus Aurelius—sported formidable beards. The Emperor Julian apparently grew one as a symbolic

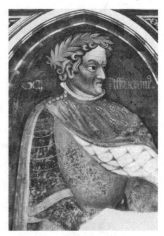

Scipio Africanus fresco by Gentile da Fabriano, Giants Room; Trinci Palace, Foligno, Italy.

repudiation of Christianity. (The early Christian church started to regulate the facial hair of its followers as a symbolic means of spiritual, and testicular, control. In the centuries that followed, as we will see, a beard could be deemed godly or satanic, depending on papal or clerical whims.)

Arab proverb: A man without a mustache is like a cat without a tail.

Commodus (161–192 CE), also known as the Idle Emperor, apparently had so much time on his hands that he brought back routine shaving. Until the last emperor of the Western Roman Empire, Romulus Augustus, all of the Roman rulers were clean shaven. Odoacer, a

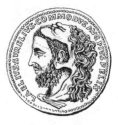

Germanic chieftain who deposed Romulus and proclaimed himself king, started a mustache fad which, as far as we can tell, has never completely disappeared—and what is now Italy remains a mo-friendly nation today.

The Teutonic conquerors of Spain, Britain, and northern Italy wore ferocious mustaches and / or beards. These Nordic barbarians more than offended their clean-shaven Romano-Christian counterparts. Not surprising then that some Christians came to view both the mustache and the beard as a mark of the beast.

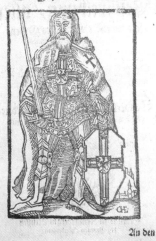

Woodcut illustration of the dress of a Hochmeister or Grand Master of the Teutonic Knights, a German Catholic military (and initially hospitaller) order founded in the 12th century.

THE MO IN MEDIEVAL AND EARLY MODERN EUROPE

We have few reliable records on hairstyles from the Dark Ages, and thus must rely on approximations of artists from later eras. The "barbarian" Gauls, Goths, Franks, and Saxons all favored long staches and shaven chins. Often the head was shaved too, except for a long tress down the back. This was serious business. To cut the hair of a Frankish king's son was to exclude him from succession. The Gaulish aristocracy wore long mustaches dyed red, which drooped down both sides of their mouths. The Celts favored long hair with their staches, but one Celtic tribe was known as the Lombards, or the long beards. Theodoric the Great, King of the Ostrogoths (454–526 CE), was sometimes shown on coins and royal stamps sporting a splendid stache. By his decree, his own descendants—Louis the Pious, Lothar I, and Louis the German—all maintained their proud military mo's to distinguish themselves from the Romans and to remember their past. Their staches represented power and a sort of follicular middle ground. The kings of the Merovingians, a Frankish dynasty (476–750 CE), wore long hair and beards dusted with gold and adorned with jewels, which resembled a facial Christmas tree. Luck was bestowed by being allowed to touch the king's beard or with a gift of a single hair from it. Throughout the sixth and seventh centuries, only slaves remained clean-shaven and bald (without a mustache in sight).

In the early Middle Ages, many men wore their hair and beards long. Short cropped hair was a sign of subservience, that is, of being both Romanized and Christianized. In western Europe, the Carolingian dynasty (750–887 CE) accepted this style and imposed it on others. While Charlemagne ordered his courtiers clean shaven, he himself wore a long mustache, demonstrating unparalleled French, or at least Frankish, chic thereafter. He wore short hair but cultivated his mustache to honor his Germanic heritage.

In the *Chanson du Roland* (written in the late eleventh century), Charlemagne is made to swear by his beard and mustache, even though he didn't always have chin whiskers and favoured the mo.

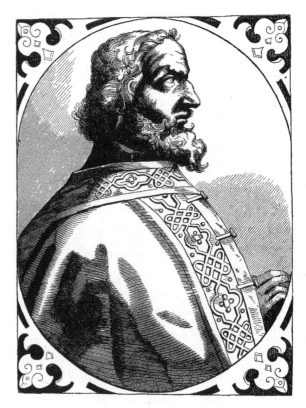

Portrait of Charlemagne *avec barbe*, facsimilie of an engraving at the end of the 16th century.

MAGYAR MO'S: A SHORT HISTORY

Hungarians have long embraced the mustache. This goes back to the days of Árpád (ca. 840–907), generally thought of as the forefather of Hungarians, the gloriously stached leader who defeated the Bulgars, the Avars, and the Goths.

William the Conqueror, Duke of Normandy (ca.1028–1087), did not wear a beard before his conquest of France, but he and his followers adopted the style soon after. During the Conquest, a few Normans and crusaders had gone beardless, but sometimes maintained a fierce military mustache. In 1096 the Archbishop of Rouen, in a fit of pique, threatened excommunication for anyone with a bearded face.

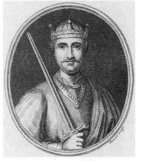

William I of England.

This made barbers in the region, who had first established a guild in France just two years earlier, very happy. Priests were sometimes allowed to have beards, only later to be told that they were forbidden; at various times, both beards and mustaches were thought to interfere with the taking of communion, as particles of the Eucharist might be entrapped in the hair.

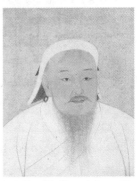

Genghis Khan, ink on silk, National Palace Museum, Taipei.

In another part of the globe at this time, the very "un-Christian" Genghis Khan (ca. 1162–1227) wore a very distinctive Fu Manchu type mustache, as did his grandson, Kublai Khan. For them, the stache was seen as a sign of wisdom, leadership, and unparalleled military might.

At about the same time but with much less gravitas, the Welsh were singing the praises of the mustache for its usefulness as an effective sieve for drink. In the fourteenth century, the Black Prince (1330–76), son of Edward III of England, is shown in portraits with a rather proud mo.

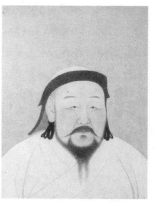

Kublai Khan, 1294, ink on silk, National Palace Museum, Taipei.

Inexplicably, in 1447 during the reign of Henry VI in England,

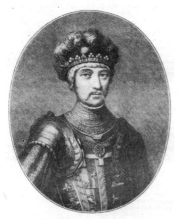

Edward the Black Prince, *Cassell's History of England*, ca. 1902.

a parliamentary decree was issued which forbade the wearing of a mustache and required that the upper lip be shaven at least every two weeks. Why did Henry have such a hate-on for the mustache? We have no record. Perhaps he viewed it as too French (i.e., the mark of a foreigner), or maybe he couldn't grow one himself. We know that he was bossy and used to getting his way. Another example of arbitrary fur-phobia occurred in 1462 when the Duke of Burgundy was obliged to shave his head for medical reasons. Five hundred of his noblemen followed suit, despite a widespread fashion for long hair at the time. (And we thought fashion lemmings were a modern phenomenon!)

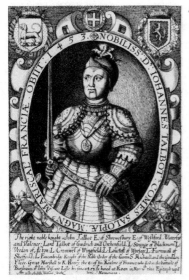

"Every Irishman must keep his upper lip shaved, or else be used as an Irish enemy."
—John Talbot, the Earl of Shrewsbury, 1447

John Talbot E: of Shrewsbury, ca. 1625–1632, engraving, British Museum, London.

During the Reformation, men grew beards to protest against the clean-shaven papists in Rome. Elizabethans ridiculed the mustache as a sign of villainy and thievery (and perhaps, "Frenchness," an even greater sin). To wear a mustache alone meant that you were a foe, fop, foreigner, or fiend. The stache was thus an immediate visual signifier that you were "other"—a mo-phobic theme that sadly recurs throughout history.

"For the more he contemplates his mustachios, the more his mind will cherish and be animated by masculine and courageous notions."
—*Elements of Education*, 1640

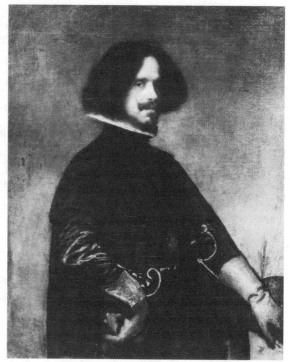

Diego Velásquez, *Self-portrait*, ca. 1645, oil on canvas, Collezione degli. Autoritratti, Firenze.

The Spanish painter Diego Velasquez (1599–1660) had a special leather case made to preserve the shape and form of his large mustache. This device became all the rage, and the fad rapidly spread to France, where the mustache was protected by law. The Spanish mustache later became an emblem of freedom and national pride.

Across the pond, the young, wig-wearing Louis XIV had a mustache, but shaved it off in 1680 when the appearance of gray whiskers betrayed his age. This act of regal vanity killed the popularity of the stache for some time in France because, of course, every loyal subject was expected to follow suit. By the seventeenth century, Charles II of England (1630–85), a historic champion of stachedom, maintained his suave, pencil-thin mustache, which many courtiers promptly copied. In general, wigs were the big fashion during this era, often worn with a pencil-thin mustache. But facial hair, including the stache, all but vanished in Europe after 1640, at least for a time (except in Turkey and Hungary, where it has never gone out of style). This again illustrates the fickle role of fads and fate on follicular expression. For example, in Russia, Peter the Great (1682–1725) attempted to make his empire more westernized by ordering his nobles and the bourgeoisie to cut off their beards and mustaches or face stiff penalties (even though he hypocritically wore a stache himself). For noblemen, gentlemen, and merchants of his capital city, St. Petersburg, there was a beard tax of 100 rubles per year, paid at the city gate in exchange for a small copper disc or beard license.

Paul Delaroch, Peter 1 of Russia, 1838, oil on canvas.

The men of the eighteenth century seemed to shun beards and mustaches altogether, though silly looking periwigs abounded. Mo's were worn only in isolated cases by the old, mad, or

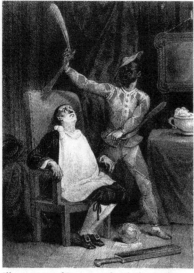

Illustration of Beaumarchais' *The Barber of Seville*, 19th century.

clueless. In 1745, barbers were no longer able to act as surgeons and dentists; an act of parliament, which received the sanction of the king, dissolved the association. It was during the eighteenth century that barbers acquired rather sinister reputations as cheats and pimps. The beard and mustache were thought to conceal men's faces, thus protecting the identity of criminals. Arthur Schopenhauer (1788–1860), the amply sideburned philosopher of pessimism, even suggested making a clean shave an absolute law.

The mustache, however, was preserved among the European military, where it had always maintained a stronghold. In France, for instance, soldiers wore remarkable crowbar mustaches; Hungarian military men were known to favor fine handlebars, and Swiss guards favored bushy staches. The military mo was seen as authoritative, manly, and deadly (read more about it in "The Military Mo" chapter).

THE VICTORIAN MO

The Victorian era was facial hair-friendly, particularly in England, but the nineteenth century did not start or end this way, as Susan Walton reminds us in her essay, "From Squalid Impropriety to Manly Respectability: The revival of beards, moustaches and martial values in the 1850s in England." If you visit the National Portrait Gallery in London, you will see that mid-century marks a striking visual transition between men without and with facial hair. Before then, Englishmen saw the mustache as a mark of foreignness (i.e., simply unforgivably French) or of French militarism, as it was worn by French soldiers in Prussia. The English also considered mustaches to be either feminine or barbaric (an emblem of, once again, the three f's: the fop, the foreigner, or the fiend).

Nineteenth-century novelist Alexandre Dumas created a trio of mustache icons when he penned *The Three Musketeers* in 1844.

During the Crimean War (1853–56), English military men were exposed to a variety of large power-mustaches, particularly among the Turks. When war against Russia was declared in March 1854, a new mustache and beard movement blossomed. Until then, British military men had been

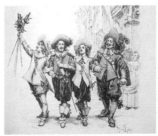

Maurice Leloir, Dumas' *The Three Musketeers*, 1894, wood engraving.

banned from wearing facial hair, but after the start of the war, the beard, mustache, and sideburns came to suggest courage, determination, and the necessary attributes of the soldier. The average man back home started to demonstrate his support of the troops by wearing the facial hair sported on the battlefield. In 1854 *The Annual Register* reported that, after some resistance, "the great mustache movement had carried its point, and hence forward the British army is to be of her suit as their continental rivals." English barbers offered special services for mustaches, which could be clipped, trimmed, pointed, curved, waxed, and made erect. When the war ended in 1856, facial hair styles of all sorts were already "in." The National Portrait Gallery becomes filled with images of ballsy mid- and late-nineteenth century leaders wearing large sideburns, thick mustaches, and very bushy beards. (Queen Victoria attempted to ban the mustache in the British navy, but the attempt was unsuccessful, and the mustache has reigned supreme on the seas ever since.) Prejudices against beards and mustaches were then forgotten for a time, and journalists repeatedly wrote about the painful act of shaving.

"There are three kinds of man you must never trust: a man who hunts south of the Thames, a man who has soup for lunch, and a man who waxes his moustache."
—Sir James Richards

Franz Josef I, Emperor of Austria, created a sensation when he allowed his sideburns to join up with his mustache; the style was named after him. However, he didn't like to be copied, and in 1838, forbade the common man from wearing the mustache and gave police the right to forcibly shave offenders.

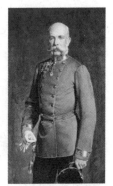

Julius von Blaas, Franz Joseph I, ca. 1923, oil on canvas.

Around the same time, a pro-hair medical argument of sorts claimed that the beard and mustache filtered the air, were protective against the elements, and could even prevent toothache and lung diseases. (Stone masons and blacksmiths, in particular, were thought to be protected from the ever-present dust and toxins of their occupations by their trademark mustaches). An absence of facial hair was now seen as unnatural, effeminate, or a sign of moral weakness. Facial hair equaled virility; Victorian gentlemen cultivated elaborate facial-hair styles, wore stylish suits and monocles, and brandished fine-cut brandy glasses. Facial hair also suggested an outdoorsy lifestyle, even while the middle class, in its manner and dress, was actually becoming more clerical, industrialized, and trapped by indoor (office) work.

The stache was a mark of imperial colonialism as well: Alfred Milner, who served in Egypt in the late nineteenth century, F.D. Lugard, a governor of Hong Kong, and Sir Richard Burton, the great explorer of Africa, all sported proud adventurer mo's. In Kenya, wild game hunter Colonel J.H. Patterson fixed his mustache into two prominent, horn-like curls, perhaps as a symbol of his hunting prowess. Jolly good!

This furry trend rapidly spread to the United States. During the American Civil War (1861–65), a facial hair style known as Burnsides became popular; this cool look—in which sideburns joined the mustache—was named after Union General Ambrose Everett Burnside. All manner of staches then took hold through the 1870s and 1880s. Mark Twain sported an unparalleled walrus mustache, and John C. Breckinridge, vice-president and Confederate general, had a fine handlebar. Soldiers in the Mexican-American War (1846–48),

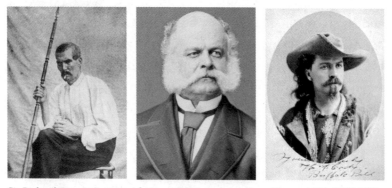

Sir Richard Francis Burton, Africa, ca. 1860, Ambrose Burnside, ca. 1865–1880, W.F. "Buffalo Bill" Cody, ca. 1875.

California gold rushers, and the grandly mustachioed William Frederick "Buffalo Bill" Cody contributed to the enduring wild-man iconography of the frontier mustache. Three US presidents—Grover Cleveland, Theodore Roosevelt, and William Taft—all had fine staches (and none has had one since). Artists began to sing the praises of the mustache on the stage and in song. Written in 1864, "If You've Only Got a Moustache" was penned by the (clean-shaven) "father of American music" Stephen Foster:

Oh! all of you poor single men,
Don't ever give up in despair,
For there's always a chance while there's life
To capture the hearts of the fair,
No matter what may be your age,
You always may cut a fine dash,
You will suit all the girls to a hair
If you've only got a moustache,
A moustache, a moustache,
If you've only got a moustache.

No matter for manners or style,
No matter for birth or for fame,
All these used to have something to do
With young ladies changing their name,
There's no reason now to despond,
Or go and do any thing rash,
For you'll do though you can't raise a cent,
If you'll only raise a moustache!
A moustache, a moustache,
If you'll only raise a moustache.

Your head may be thick as a block,
And empty as any foot-ball,
Oh! your eyes may be green as the grass
Your heart just as hard as a wall.
Yet take the advice that I give,
You'll soon gain affection and cash,
And will be all the rage with the girls,
If you'll only get a moustache,
A moustache, a moustache,
If you'll only get a moustache.

I once was in sorrow and tears
Because I was jilted you know,
So right down to the river I ran
To quickly dispose of my woe,
A good friend he gave me advice
And timely prevented the splash,
Now at home I've a wife and ten heirs,
And all through a handsome moustache,
A moustache, a moustache,
And all through a handsome moustache.

In European countries, the mustache's popularity also waxed (ahem) and waned: the King of Bavaria forbade his men to wear them in 1838, although the ban didn't last long. Throughout the early nineteenth century, French militiamen, the Hussars, and Prussian guards all wore mustaches; in time these became de rigueur for all European military men. In 1890, a Hungarian law forbade stache removal for enlisted men. The Archduke Franz Ferdinand of Austria (1863–1914) wore a trimmed and waxed walrus mustache. Spaniards and Frenchmen continued to wear their long-celebrated mustaches with national pride.

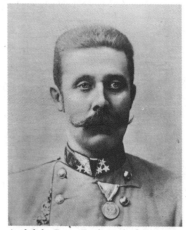

Archduke Franz Ferdinand of Austria.

The macho mustache became a standard issue for military men throughout Europe, who trimmed it, waxed it, dyed it, and made it a powerful symbol of their stature. From the nineteenth century to the middle of World War II, all ranks in the British army were actually forbidden to shave their upper lips. This stache-friendly regulation was revoked in 1916 after army men lobbied hard for the right to be clean-shaven. Nevertheless, the mustache became a badge of military rank; low-ranking officers were permitted only a tiny growth but, as they rose through the hierarchy, were allowed a bushy, showy lip shelf. Beards were not allowed, except for commanding officers. The military stache was clearly a proud status symbol (more fur = more power).

Early Mo-Phobia: In 1862, English control freak and mustache hater Henry Budd asserted in his will that if either of his sons grew a mo, they would forfeit their inheritance at once.

Britain's *Punch* magazine poked fun at the plethora of furry faces found in cities and towns across the nation. In 1854, the magazine published an article called "Reason and a Razor," which outlined the pros and cons of the beard and mustache and noted that "[g]allant captains wear moustaches—therefore some praise them. Swindlers wear moustaches to pass for gallant captains: musical professors also wear moustaches to pass for foreigners; wherefore others disparage them. This is not philosophy." By the 1860s, most respectable Victorian men wore beards, sideburns, or the mustache. Clean-shaven, smooth-talking diplomats on both sides of the pond were replaced with men of courage and determination, identifiable firstly by their facial hair.

Napoleon III (1808–73) was known to heavily wax his mustache into sharp points, in a style called the Imperial.

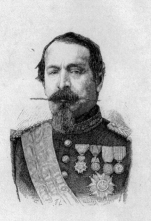

NAPOLÉON III

"The moustache should be neat and not too large, and such fopperies as cutting the points thereof or twisting them up to the fineness of needles—though patronized by the Emperor of the French—are decidedly a proof of vanity."
—The Habits of Good Society: A Handbook of Etiquette for Ladies and Gentlemen, 1859

In the late nineteenth century, an industry producing combs, brushes, waxes, oils, dyes, and hairnets burst forth to service the first, real, unstoppable mustache revolution. In 1872, a product that prevented food from being trapped in facial hair was patented, so ubiquitous were the beard, mustache, and sideburns. Stache combs and mustache cups were issued in all shapes and sizes. Toward the end of the century, a mustache trainer (sort of like a stache-bra)

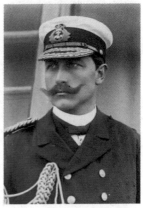

Wilhelm II of Germany, ca. 1890.

named after Kaiser Wilhelm II (1859–1951), became all the rage. Stache wearers could even buy a mustache curler with a heating apparatus. Once the mo caught fire, clever fellows came up with numerous products to keep it spiffy.

"An emphatic mustache can redeem an intractable countenance."
—Sir Robert Eric Mortimer Wheeler, archaeologist (1890–1976)

MUSTACHE CUPS

Invented in the mid-1800s, mustache cups are now sought-after collectors' items. In Victorian times, most men had impressive mustaches, many waxed and dyed, groomed and curled. When these coifed mo's came into contact with hot

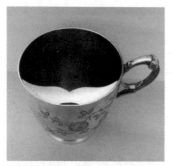

tea (which Englishmen drank in vast quantities), the mustache wax would melt and the dye would run, much to the embarassment of the stached gentlemen. As a result, clever English potter Harvey Adams created a "mustache guard," a curved ledge that went across the cup with an opening in the middle through which one could sip tea

Victorian silverplate mustache cup made by Simpson, Hall, Miller & Co., Connecticut.

while keeping the mustache and upper lip dry. This amenity became very popular and eventually made its way from England and Europe to North America. In 1901, a separate insertable mo-guard was patented in the US.

SNOODS

A snood is a gauze band that fastens across the mustache to help keep it in shape. Popular in Victorian times, it, like the Kaiser Wilhelm, was a stache-bra of sorts.

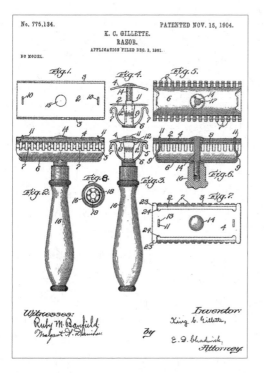

No. 775,134. PATENTED NOV. 15, 1904.

K. C. GILLETTE.

RAZOR.

APPLICATION FILED DEC. 3, 1901.

NO MODEL.

Witnesses:
Ruby M. Banfield
Margaret P. Dinnihan.

by

Inventor:
King C. Gillette,
E. D. Chadwick,
Attorney.

K.C. Gillette, front page of Gillett's razor patent, November 15, 1904.

In 1912, Fritz Baudisch patented a mustache and lip guard (patent number GB191127119), essentially an antiseptic paper disc that could be folded over the edge of any cup to keep the mo dry while its wearer slurped his drink.

But not long after the turn of the century, the British Empire-stache crashed. (The anti-fuzz movement may actually have begun in the 1890s when King Camp Gillette, who himself wore a mustache, introduced his safety razor with disposal blades.) In the early twentieth century, Americans started waging an all-out attack on the mustache. In 1903, a reporter for the *Chicago Tribune* stood on a busy corner and counted, in one hour, 3,000 men; he reported that, of these, 1,656 were clean shaven, 108 had beards, and 1,236 had mustaches. The journalist concluded that clean-shavenness was starting to sweep the nation. In the same year, *Harper's Weekly* published an article called "The Passing of Beards," a fond farewell to fur and a celebration of the clean-shaven face, which was now admired "for its honesty."

Even the medical tide was turning against the stache. In 1909, the *New York Times* published a short article entitled "Mustache Harbors Germs: Kiss Leaves Deposit of Bacilli on French Woman's Lips." Apparently, a French scientist published an experiment in which he showed that the lips of the mustached man "had colonized the lady's lips with the bacilli of tuberculosis, diphtheria, pneumonia, and numerous other unpleasant microbes." One of Britain's pre-eminent medical journals, *The Lancet*, reported that men with mustaches were actually more likely to suffer from colds; the bristles, rather than acting as air filters, actually provided a perfect medium in which nasty bugs flourished.

Christpher Oldstone-Moore in his essay, "Mustaches and Masculine Codes in Early Twentieth-Century America," reminds us that the hyper-scientific, ultra-ambitious twentieth century emphasized the prevention of disease and the promotion of public hygiene, youthfulness, discipline, and corporate ambitions. A clean-shaven face came to suggest that a man was tidy, a team player, and reliable, while the mo came to indicate quite the opposite. The new corporate ethos featured the white-collar man; he was boyish, athletic, trustworthy, and virtuous. Wearing a mustache, particularly a graying one, could hold a chap's career back. For example, by

1917, the Burlington Northern Railroad decreed that its conductors could not have facial hair. Then the police department in Evanston, Illinois, ordered its officers to shave off their mustaches. Other police departments followed suit. Women complained if their men came back from World War I with any kind of facial hair still in place, particularly the mustache, as it was now considered to be unforgivably patriarchal. Mustaches were associated with "old-country" European military might. Twentieth-century barbers, of course, were all too keen to promote the clean-cut image.

Mo' Mo-Phobia: "A civilian of great intelligence and sense would never wear a mustache."
—Charles MacLaren, editor of *The Scotsman*, 1891

Most Expensive Mo?:
Aussie cricket player Merv Hughes insured his
bushy handlebar stache in the late '80s and into
the '90s for £200,000.

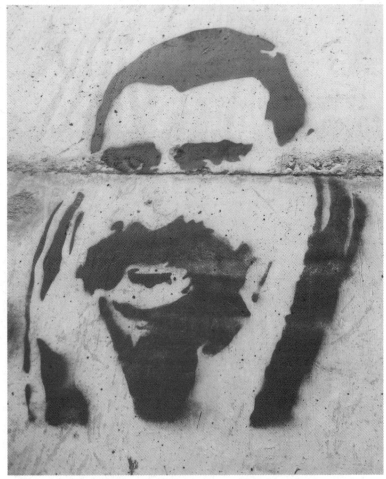

A stencil of an image of Merv Hughes in a laneway in Fitzroy, Australia.

THE MO IN MODERN TIMES

"There's a man outside with a big black mustache. Tell him I've got one." —Groucho Marx

If you grew up in the twentieth century, your take on the mustache has inevitably been shaped (and distorted) by images you've encountered repeatedly in movies, on television, and in comic books and advertising campaigns. New media and social media in the twenty-first century allow even greater and swifter propagation of images, stylistic innovations, flash-fads, and unexamined stereotypes and cultural projections associated with facial hair.

Prominent twentieth-century mustachioed figures can help us interpret how the stache was defined (and in some instances, demeaned) as the century progressed. Conjure up images of Groucho Marx with his bushy eyebrows and walrus mustache; Joseph Stalin and Adolf Hitler with their fascist

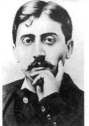

Marcel Proust, 1900.

fur; Chester Conklin as a bumbling Keystone Kop; villains in B-movie melodramas sporting Fu Manchus; barbershop quartets complete with straw hats, striped jackets, and classic handlebar mustaches; Salvador Dali and Marcel Proust with their matchless artistic mustaches; and Albert Einstein with his frizzy gray hair and furry lip—the epitome of eccentric scientific genius—and you will see how

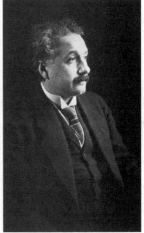

Albert Einstein, 1921.

the stache has come to be associated with so many of the most famous and familiar faces we've known in the last hundred years.

TRADEMARK MUSTACHES: MO'S INCREASE SALES!

In the world of advertising, if you find an iconic product mascot, you've got it made. The following ad campaigns have recruited furry fellows that are cuddly, cute, culinarily gifted, culturally stereotyped, or mucho macho, to shill products of all kinds.

- The Brawny Man: a character created in 1974 for Brawny paper towels
- The Man in the Hathaway Shirt: 1950s shirt campaign for C.F. Hathaway
- The Camel Man 1970s–'80s cigarette campaign
- Mr. Whipple: Charmin toilet paper, 1964–85
- Got Milk?: ad campaign featuring men and women wearing jaunty milk mustaches; launched in 1993 and still running
- Juan Valdez: romantic spokesman in coffee ads, created by the National Federation of Colombian Coffee Growers in 1959
- Julius Pringles: the face of Pringles potato chips
- Cap'n Crunch, a.k.a. Horatio Magellan Crunch: breakfast cereal mascot
- Chef Boyardee, formerly Chef Boy-Ar-Dee: tinned pasta icon
- The Frito Bandito: character in Fritos ads who was, for a time, synonymous with corn chips

THE HOLLYWOOD MO—FROM SUSPECT TO SOPHISTICATE

From the earliest days of cinema, Hollywood's popular mustached figures, including Charlie Chaplin's lovable but hapless Tramp, created in 1914, gave a comic aura to the mo. In the 1920s, pencil-thin mustaches appeared on the faces of villains in films (think of poor Nell being tied to the railroad tracks by a mustachioed fiend in a black cape). Ronald Colman and Douglas Fairbanks, Sr. grew them as indicators of debonair sophistication. By the '30s, Clark Gable and Douglas Fairbanks, Jr. had trademark mustaches that made them top romantic leads. Gable became known as the king of Hollywood in large part due to his trademark stache. As Rhett Butler in *Gone with the Wind*, his mustache suggested virility,

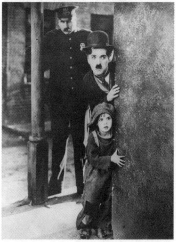

Publicity photo from Charlie Chaplin's 1921 movie *The Kid*.

aggression, self-centeredness, and swagger, which imbued the mustache with layer upon layer of new meaning. (Even the usually clean-shaven Bing Crosby grew a mustache for one of his films in 1935, a musical called *Mississippi*.)

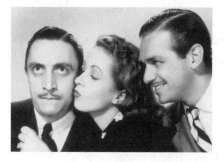

Publicity photo from *The Rage of Paris*, 1938. (left to right) Mischa Auer, Danielle Darrieux, & Douglas Fairbanks, Jr.

"Don't think I don't know who's been spreading gossip about me... After all the nice things I've said about that hag. When I get hold of her, I'll tear out every hair of her moustache!"
—Tallulah Bankhead on Bette Davis

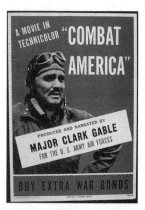

Clark Gable on the poster of the movie *Combat America*, 1941.

Mustaches were particularly popular in England in the '30s and were given names such as the Consort, the Shadow, Major General, Guardsman, Captain, and Regent. (See these styles in the Appendix)

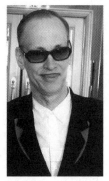

John Waters in Cannes, 2007. Photo, Alain Zirah.

"My signature look is my mustache. I grew it when I was nineteen in honor of Little Richard. I trim it every day. I use a throwaway razor on the top, cuticle scissors on the bottom, and I fill it in with a pencil. I'm so used to it, I can do it blindfolded." —John Waters in *The Guardian*, December 11, 2010.

In 1930s Hollywood, "Women would not appear in public without their make-up. Homosexuals would not appear without their 'beards.' Heterosexual men would not appear in public without their mustaches."

—Stephen Colbert, *I Am America (And So Can You!)*

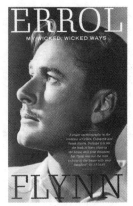

Actor Errol Flynn (1909–1959).

THE GREATEST MUSTACHES IN FILM: A QUIZ

Films have deeply informed our interpretation of the mustachioed face. It all started with stache-twirling villains, then moved to the comical anti-hero and the debonair and action-seeking leading man. How well do you know your cinematic stache? Match these famous actors to their movies:

1. Douglas Fairbanks
   (1883–1939)

2. Chester Conklin
   (1886–1971)

3. Charlie Chaplin
   (1889–1977)

4. Julius Henry
   "Groucho" Marx
   (1890–1977)

5. Ronald Charles
   (1891–1958)

6. Clark Gable
   (1901–1960)

7. Errol Flynn
   (1909–1959)

8. David Niven
   (1910–1983)

9. Charles Bronson
   (1921–2003)

10. Lee Van Cleef
    (1925–1989)

11. Robert Goulet
    (1933–2007)

12. Burt Reynolds
    (1936–)

13. Billy Dee Williams
    (1937–)

14. Richard Pryor
    (1940–2005)

15. Richard Roundtree
    (1942–)

16. Sam Elliott (1944–)

17. Cheech Marin
    (1946–)

18. Eddie Murphy
    (1961–)

19. Sacha Baron Cohen
    (1971–)

A. *Borat*

B. *Brigadoon*

C. *Captain Blood*

D. *Coming to America*

E. *Deliverance*

F. *Duck Soup*

G. *Gone with the Wind*

H. *Keystone Kops*

I. *Robin Hood*

J. *Shaft*

K. *Superman III*

L. *A Double Life*

M. *The Empire Strikes Back*

N. *The Good, the Bad and the Ugly*

O. *The Lion King*

P. *The Magnificent Seven*

Q. *The Pink Panther*

R. *The Tramp*

S. *We Were Soldiers*

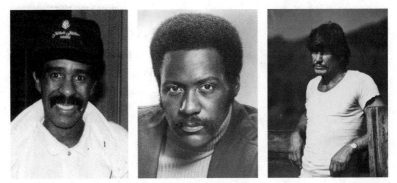

Richard Pryor, Alan Light photo, 1986. Richard Roundtree, publicity photo from TV series *Shaft*, 1973. Charles Bronson, Fish Cop at en.wikipedia, 1973.

Answers: 1-I; 2-H; 3-R; 4-F; 5-L; 6-G; 7-C; 8-Q; 9-P; 10-N; 11-B; 12-E; 13-M; 14-K; 15-J; 16-S; 17-O; 18-D; 19-A

The Porn-stache: Ron Jeremy, star of 2,000 XXX films, is the son of a physicist father and editor mother, and this mo icon has a theater degree. John Holmes, the 1970s XXX actor known for his massive appendage, was the first famous stached porn star.

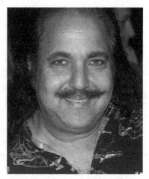

Ron Jeremy, 2005. Photo, lukeisback.com.

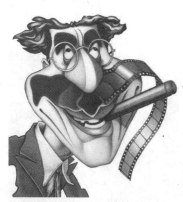

Caricature of Groucho Marx by Greg Williams.

Groucho Marx initially glued on a stache in his vaudeville days or used greasepaint until he grew his own mo to match his ultra-thick eyebrows.

THE MID-CENTURY MO

By the 1940s, perhaps in response to some highly sinister mustaches that gained notoriety in World War II, most actors had abandoned the mo altogether. Journalist Edith

Efron, writing in the *New York Times Sunday Magazine* in 1944 summed up the mustache as follows: "it plays many roles today. It is Chaplin pathetic, Hitler psychopathic, Gable debonair, and Lou Lehr wacky. It perplexes, it fascinates, it amuses, and it repels." The stache had once again become

"iffy." As a response, in 1947, English actor Jimmy Edwards established the Handlebar Club in a London pub, to show that "men with moustaches are men of good character." Similar clubs soon sprang up across Europe (see "Champions of the Modern Mustache Movement" in the Appendix). But despite such efforts, the stache continued to go downhill in the next decade. Men coming home from World War

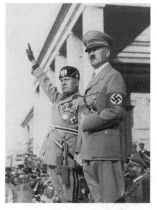

Adolf Hitler (1889–1945).

II adopted the clean-shaven look as they became educated under the G.I. Bill, pursued middle-class professions, and captured the American dream. The culture was still reeling

from the war, and any potential associations to Hitler (including stylistic ones) were to be avoided. Although the Zapata stache, named after Emiliano Zapata, guerrilla leader of the 1917 Mexican Revolution, caught on for a while (after Marlon Brando played him in the 1956 film *Viva Zapata!*), the mainstream majority in the 1950s saw the beatniks—who were goateed and mustached, and fancied berets and poetry readings—as a fringe element.

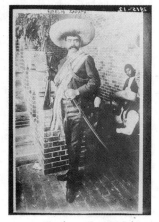

Emiliano Zapata Salazar (1879–1919).

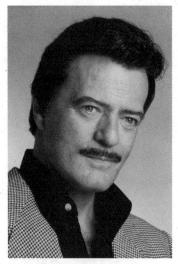

Robert Goulet (1933–2007), courtesy of the Estate of Robert Goulet.

In the swinging '60s a facial-hair boom included the return of the stache—as long as it didn't look militaristic (for "make love not war" reasons). The mo's come-back was so great in this decade that the Kent Brushes company (established in 1777 in England) reissued a long-shelved mustache brush. Actors such as Robert Goulet perpetuated the celebrity stache as a symbol of seductive masculinity, later emulated by stars like Burt Reynolds. The Beatles, the ultimate trendsetters of the decade, all sported mustaches at some point and occasionally all at the same time (e.g., the 1967 *Sgt Peppers Lonely Hearts Club Band* album cover). The hippie movement saw the further flowering of all forms of facial fur,

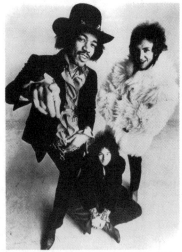

including classic staches (and big hair) on well-known personalities as diverse as Jimi Hendrix and David Crosby, Frank Zappa and Jerry Rubin.

Another furry classic, the gay mustache, appeared in 1970s personified by the Village People who in turn were inspired by the ultra-macho San Fran clones, who wore construction boots, tight jeans, bomber jackets, and well-groomed mustaches. The

Promotional photo of The Jimi Hendrix Experience, 1968.

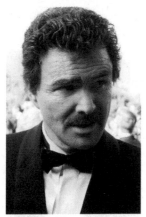

Burt Reynolds at the 43rd Annual Emmy Awards. Photo, Alan Light.

'70s also saw the growing popularity of gay, straight, and bisexual pornographic films in which male actors wore the point stache. Some critics believe that the evolution of the mustache into a gay, bi, or swinger signifier explained its near disappearance in the '80s and '90s. Was this due to the culture's homophobia or to the fact that men did not want their mustachioed faces (and hence their sexual orientation) misread?

In these same decades, however, certain celebrities' mustaches were almost as famous as they were, including those of actor Burt Reynolds, Olympic swimming champion Mark Spitz, legal eagle Alan Dershowitz, singer Stevie Wonder, media magnate Ted Turner, film critic Gene Shalit, *Magnum, P.I.* star Tom Selleck, and Canadian singer (with The Guess Who) Burton Cummings. All were known to at least temporarily repackage themselves without lip fuzz, perhaps in search of a more youthful look, but most wisely re-grew their trademark mustaches before too long.

In the 1990s, any man with a stache stood out in a landscape barren of lip fur. The exception to this rule was the emergence of a playful

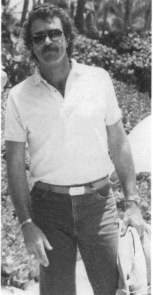

Tom Selleck on the set of the TV series *Magnum P.I.*, 1984. Photo, Alan Light.

artistic trend in which graffiti artists the world over sprayed mustaches onto all kinds of advertising images, and this was followed by the very popular milk promotion campaign "Got Milk?" in which well-known personalities are shown sporting a "milk-stache." At the end of the 1990s, only some ten million American men were thought to be wearing mustaches. But with the emergence of charity movements such as Movember (see Appendix, p.140), men began to rediscover the endless fun of the stache: it could be waxed, dyed, twirled, or dipped into various sauces prior to kissing. By the end of the twentieth century, perhaps as a nod to irony, young men on college campuses started growing a variety of mo's, from Fu Manchus to pencil-thins, and from porn-staches to walruses.

A Documentary Mo: Morgan Spurlock rose to fame in February 2004 when he gorged on McDonald's food, gained twenty-five pounds, and let his mustache do the talking in his documentary *Super Size Me*; alas, he is now without it. His latest film, 2012's *Mansome*, features a discussion of facial hair in the history of men's grooming that includes an interview with, ahem, the author of this very book!

GREATEST MUSTACHES ON TELEVISION

Television has done much to shape public opinion about the stache. From the musical to the whimsical and from the nerdy to the dashing, here is a list of the greatest mustaches that have appeared on tv:

- John Astin (Gomez Addams on *The Addams Family*)
- Sonny Bono (*The Sonny and Cher Comedy Hour*)
- Walt Disney (animated empire-builder)
- Dennis Franz (*NYPD Blue*)
- Sherman Helmsley (*The Jeffersons*)
- Christopher Hewett (*Mr. Belvedere*)
- Hulk Hogan (World Wrestling Federation wrestler)
- Gabriel Kaplan (*Welcome Back, Kotter*)
- Bob Keeshan (*Captain Kangaroo*)
- Hal Linden (*Barney Miller*)
- Dr Phil McGraw (TV talk show therapist)
- Rob Reiner (*All in the Family*)
- Dan Rowan (*Rowan & Martin's Laugh-In*)
- Geraldo Rivera (entertainment journalist)
- Tom Selleck (*Magnum, P.I.*)
- Gene Shalit (film reviewer)
- Dick Smothers (*The Smothers Brothers Comedy Hour*)
- John Stossel (*20/20* host)
- Alex Trebek (*Jeopardy* host; now clean-shaven)
- Guy Williams (*Zorro*)

Superheroes never have mustaches. Supervillains sometimes do. But the creator of some of the best characters in both categories, Marvel's Stan Lee, wears a proud mo!

CARTOON AND COMIC BOOK MUSTACHES

No compilation of television mustaches would be complete without a list of cartoon characters, who run the gamut from furry to friendly to fiendish. Many of your own projections, associations, and unexamined biases about the stache likely come from the endless hours that

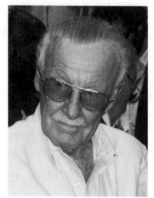

Stan Lee at the 2011 New York Comic Con. Photo, Luigi Novi.

you spent as a child, when you were at your most impressionable, watching these fellows on television or reading about their adventures in comic books.

- Asterix and Obelix (*The Adventures of Asterix*)
- Big Gay Al (*South Park*)
- Boris Badenov (*The Rocky and Bullwinkle Show*)
- Bruce the Performance Artist, Carter Pewterschmidt, Cleveland Brown, and Tom Tucker (*Family Guy*)
- Captain Hook (*Peter Pan*)
- Chief Inspector Jacques Clouseau (*The Pink Panther*)
- Clo-Clo (*The Adventures of Nero*)

- Dick Dastardly (*Wacky Races*)
- The Lorax (Dr Seuss's *The Lorax*)
- Mario and Luigi (*Super Mario Brothers*)
- Ming the Merciless (*Flash Gordon*)
- Mister Geppetto (*The Adventures of Pinocchio*)
- Monty (*Chip 'n' Dale: Rescue Rangers*)
- Mr Potato Head (*Toy Story*)
- Ned Flanders (*The Simpsons*)
- Ringmaster (*Dumbo*)
- Snidely Whiplash (*Dudley Do-Right*)
- Mr Spacely (*The Jetsons*)
- Thomson and Thompson (*The Adventures of Tintin*)
- J. Wellington Wimpy (*Popeye*)
- Yosemite Sam (*Looney Toons*)

Mario, the lovable Super Mario Brothers video game star, first took a jump in 1981. Mario had a big head, a big stache, and a red hat, because his creator for Nintendo, Mr Miyamoto, did not have the technical means to make the character's hair or facial features move properly.

HO-MO MASCULINITIES

Throughout history, men who loved men wore the same kinds of mustaches (or beards or clean-shaven mugs) as their straight counterparts, following social, class, and style norms. As a homosexual, in more arduous times, the last thing you wanted to do was stand out (although Oscar Wilde had the élan to shave when all of his stodgy Victorian counterparts were furry). This changed in the 1970s when San Francisco's Castro-district gay boys entrenched the mo as part of their homo macho uniform. The stache has been read by many as gay, bi, or swinging ever since.

"They [homosexuals] have already claimed mustaches and short-shorts. They've ruined them for all the rest of us ... Mustaches don't make you gay, but they don't help." —Stephen Colbert, Comedy Central's *Colbert Report*, **broadcast January 30, 2008**

A HISTORY OF GAY AND BI STACHES

Check out this random sampling of splendid homo-mo's!

- Edward Albee (1928–): US playwright; author of *Who's Afraid of Virginia Woolf?*
- C.P. Cavafy (1863–1933): Homoerotic Greek poet
- Erasmus (1466–1536): Dutch Renaissance humanist
- Rainer Werner Fassbinder (1945–1982): German film director
- Count Adelsward Fersen (1880–1923): Swedish count who had a pink mass on his gay wedding day

- Errol Flynn (1909–1959): Sometimes-mustachioed bi film star

- E.M. Forster (1879–1970): Author of *Maurice*, a tender boy-meets-boy story

- John Galliano (1960–): Disgraced fashion designer

- Horatio Herbert, Lord Kitchener (1850–1916): English colonel and poster boy for military recruitment

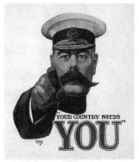

Lord Kitchener calls upon British citizens to enlist for the First World War, 1914.

- John Maynard Keynes (1883–1946): British economist

- William Somerset Maugham (1874–1965): Novelist, author of (non-S/M classic) *Of Human Bondage*

- Armistead Maupin (1944–): Novelist; author *Tales of the City* series

- Freddie Mercury (1946–1991): British musician, lead singer of Queen

- Marcel Proust (1871–1922): Aesthete and author of *In Search of Lost Time*

- George Santayana (1863–1952): Philosopher, poet, and novelist

- Harry Stack Sullivan (1892–1949): Distinguished US psychoanalyst

- Village People (formed in 1977): Randy Jones (The Cowboy); Glenn Hughes (The Leatherman); David "Scar" Hodo (The Cop); Alex Briley (The GI) who showed the power of the "gay stache"

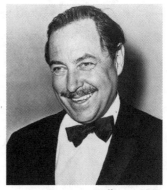

Tennessee Williams, 1965.

- John Waters (1946–): film director of *Pink Flamingos* and *Hairspray*
- Clifton Webb (1889–1966): Stage and early movie actor
- Tennessee Williams (1911–1983): Southern US playwright; author of *A Streetcar Named Desire*

The Trans-stache Drag kings and female-to-male (FTM) transsexuals have long known the emblematic, instantaneously virilizing power of the mustache. Check out our favorite trans-staches on Youtube and Facebook: "Fake Mustache Drag King Troupe" and "The Drag King Show" (Calgary, Alberta). For a superb FTM mustache how-to grow-guide, go to *ftmguide.org/facialhair.html*.

THE ROCK 'N' ROLL MUSTACHE PANTHEON

Maybe rock stars have embraced the mustache to such a great extent because they can "push the envelope" more easily than others and don't have to account to anyone but their fans. In online polls, Freddie Mercury usually comes out on top (as it were) as the all-time rock-mo favorite. This list may be alphabetical, but we're still putting Freddie first!

- Freddie Mercury (Queen)
- Duane Allman (Allman Brothers Band)
- Frank Beard (ZZ Top)
- The Beatles

- Chuck Berry

- David Crosby (Crosby, Stills and Nash)

- Burton Cummings (The Guess Who)

- Jimi Hendrix

- Lemmy Kilmister (Motörhead)

- Little Richard

- Phil Lynott (Thin Lizzy)

- John Oates (Hall & Oates)

- Axl Rose (Guns N' Roses)

- Derek Smalls (of Spinal Tap, as portrayed by Harry Shearer)

- The Village People

- Stevie Wonder

- Frank Zappa (The Mothers of Invention)

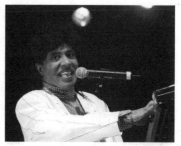

Little Richard performing at the University of Texas Forty Acres Festival in 2007.

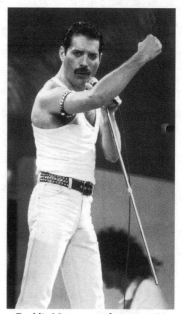

Freddie Mercury performing at Live Aid, 1985. Photo, Peter Still.

Freddie Mercury first revealed his fabulous mo in June 1980 in the video for "Play the Game."

> **"Oh, I wish I had a pencil thin mustache, / Then I could solve some mysteries too."**
> **—Jimmy Buffett, "Pencil Thin Mustache"**

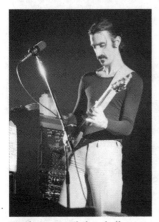

In 2008, Gail Zappa, widow of Frank, sued a German rock festival for the unauthorized use of her husband's name—and the image of his stache and soul patch. She lost the suit in 2009.

Frank Zappa, Ekeberghallen, Oslo, Norway, 1977.

Having reviewed the many cultural references triggered by the mo' listed above, pause for a moment and ask: Which Stache Am I?

bandit	cab driver
barbarian	cad
barbershop quartet singer	cartoon villain
baseball hero	clown
bellhop	composer
biker	confederate soldier
buffoon	cop

Cossack

cowboy

detective

dictator

duffer

fashion model

fireman

fop

gangster

gay/bi dude

geek

gigolo

gold rush prospector

grandpa

hippie

hipster

horseman

lion-tamer

macho man

Mafioso

magician

maharajah

matador

musketeer

outlaw

painter

patriot

pawnbroker

perpetual virgin

pervert

philanthropist

pimply teenager

poet

politico

porn star

product pitchman

rock star

safari enthusiast

scientific genius

spy

strip club announcer

strongman

suave thespian

swashbuckler

swinger

terrorist

trendsetter

trucker

vaudevillian

Victorian gent

villain

waiter

warmonger

wild man

wrestler

all of the above?

> **"In the old days villains had moustaches and kicked the dog. Audiences are smarter today."**
> **—Alfred Hitchcock**

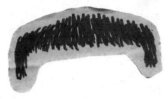

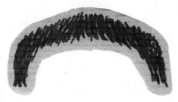

Clockwise from top;
Paul McCartney, George
Harrison, Ringo Starr,
John Lennon.

In 1967, the Beatles wore mo's on the cover of *Sgt. Pepper's Lonely Hearts Club Band* and enclosed cardboard staches within. Paul McCartney explained his Sgt. Pepper stache as a pragmatic response to a tumble from a moped in 1966; the mo hid his swollen lip!

NO STACHE WITHOUT THE RAZOR: A HISTORY OF SHAVING

Any history of the mustache naturally implies a parallel history of shaving, as no stache would shine without an otherwise shorn mug. The god Mercury was said to have invented the razor, but credit for hair removal actually goes to the much less glamorous. We may think of Stone-Agers as universally fuzzy, but by 100,000 BCE, primitives enjoyed filing teeth, tattooing the body, and using seashells to pluck out hair. The first disposable razors—made of sharp flint—appeared around 30,000 BCE; they must have been wretchedly painful to use. Why some prehistoric men removed their facial hair and/or kept a stache, given the inconvenience and agony, is open to speculation. Perhaps the shorn were required to demonstrate submissiveness to their leaders, or maybe Wilma and Betty simply preferred smoother kisses. Iron blades first appeared around 1000 BCE.

By 300 BCE, Egyptians took the whole shaving trend to heart, as they resolutely believed that head, facial, and body hair were animalistic and uncivilized. Priests shaved not only their heads and facial hair, but also their entire bodies at least once every three days; hieroglyphic records describe these grooming techniques. Wealthy Egyptians, some of whom wore mustaches, kept full-time barbers on staff, but for those less rich and in need of a shave, specific street corners bristled (as it were) with barber shops. Razors became more elaborate—gold-plated, engraved, encrusted with jewels—and were buried (as we discover when we desecrate tombs) with royalty. Any enduring stone images of the hirsute from that time represent peasants, madmen, slaves, or, not surprisingly, what were later called barbarians (most of whom had mustaches).

By 500 BCE, Alexander the Great insisted that his troops shave to avoid dangerous beard-grabbing in combat, and because he believed it looked tidier. His logic persisted for almost two centuries. In Rome, the rich retained servants to shave them, while the less wealthy would head to a barber who used an iron *novacila*, a shaving instrument which tended to rust and grow blunt, cutting many and killing a few with tetanus.

In 296 BCE, the Greek entrepreneur Publicus Ticinus Maenas (or so the story goes) imported professional barbers from Sicily to Rome, which meant that shaving became even trendier. As is still the case, young men ritualized their first shave, usually at the age of about twenty-one (late bloomers compared to today); they used iron blades with long handles. Friends and elders were invited to witness the procedure and to bring elaborate gifts. The shorn tufts were then gathered in gold or silver boxes to be presented to the gods.

Julius Caesar had his beard hairs plucked out individually with tweezers. This was considerably more time-consuming, but no doubt safer than entrusting his regal throat to the blade of a corruptible servant. Meanwhile, his soldiers were stuck with rubbing their beards and mustaches off with pumice stones. The Greco-Roman world remained clean-shaven until the Emperor Hadrian (76–138 CE) grew a beard to hide either a bad

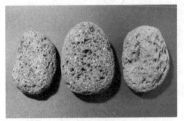

Pumice stones from the beach of the island of Stromboli, Sicily, Italy. Photo, Norbert Nagel, 2011.

case of acne, facial warts, or scars, depending on your source. Young men followed their leader, and as a result facial hair sprouted defiantly on Roman faces once again for several centuries.

In the Middle Ages in Europe, the grooming industry was booming—cosmetics, deodorants, teeth cleaners, and the like became popular among the nobility. It could be argued that there were religious reasons for this fastidiousness after the Great Schism in 1054 between the Eastern Orthodox and the Roman Catholic Church. Western clergy insisted on shaven faces so that Catholics could be distinguished not only from their lapsed counterparts, but also from so-called "infidels" such as Muslims and Jews. In these centuries, a lone mustache was often seen as the "sign of the Beast."

Shaving continued to be somewhat of a treacherous operation until well into the seventeenth century when a smooth face under a wigged head was de rigueur. In 1680, a type of folding razor first appeared in England. Frenchman Jean Jacques Perret conceptualized the

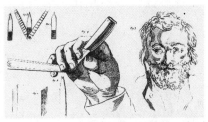

Drawing from the 1770 book of Jean-Jacques Perret, *La pogonotomie, ou L'art d'apprendre a se raser soi-meme.*

first safety razor around 1770, which had a wooden guard along the blade. He also wrote an early self-help book entitled *La Pogonotomie (The Art of Learning to Shave Oneself)*. The Perret razor was eventually manufactured and its use became widespread in the late 1700s. The invention of cast steel had occurred along some years earlier, in 1740, and it proved very useful for razor-making.

Mo Medical Trivia: In the 1880s, Frenchmen anointed their mustaches with carbolic acid to prevent cholera.

The French, ever inventive and devout mustache wearers, also introduced the shaving brush in 1748. These were often fashioned from stiff badger hair, which made shaving more pleasurable and convenient, as applying soap to the face before shaving it softened the whiskers. Thus began the link between shaving and luxurious pampering that we continue

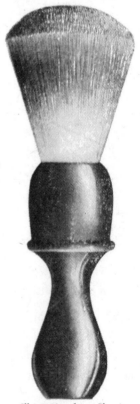

Illustration from *Shaving Made Easy*, 1905.

to embrace today. Most European men continued to be shaved by professional barbers until about 1900. (Eighteenth-century French philosopher Jean-Jacques Rousseau, however, lamented the effeminacy of the shaven face, suggesting that men and women should "no more be alike in mind than in face," in *Emile: Or On Education*, published in 1762.)

Shaving, grooming, fussing, and preening all became the rage in London in the 1800s, thanks largely to a major fop named Beau Brummell, who dedicated his life to being a fashionable gent, shaving several times a day and coiffing his hair in three parts. Sadly, he accrued huge gambling debts and fled to France in 1816 where he eventually died in an asylum, much less stylish, penniless, and insane. Our enduring (and closed-minded) suspicion of the over-groomed, foppish male can be linked to Brummel's sad fate.

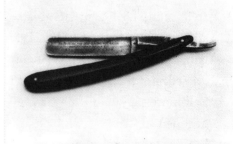

John Barrymore

"Beau Brummel"

Beau Brummel, film poster, 1924.

Meanwhile, Brummel's contemporary, the brilliant and infinitely more practical scientist Michael Faraday, found a way to add silver to steel razor blades, rendering them sharper and less prone to rust. Straight steel or cut-throat razors were manufactured in Sheffield, England; their blades were laboriously forged one-by-one by skilled metal workers. Self-grooming was becoming a huge market and technology its ever humble servant. A striking innovation occurred in 1847 when another Englishman invented a razor with the blade perpendicular to the handle. The so-called "hoe razor" was easier to hold and to maneuver and remains an enduring design.

Example of a straight razor, manufactured by Geo Wostenholm & Son, Sheffield, England. Photo, Brandi Sims, 2009.

But the popularity of shaving waned again during the Victorian beard and mustache boom, when beards and staches ruled Britannia. Victorian gents in all their macho glory were nonetheless great consumers of scents, soaps, and mustache waxes and dyes, produced to keep all furry matters in check. Various English treatises described beard shaving as effeminate, unnatural, irrational, unmanly, and ungodly. Scottish purists in particular condemned Sunday shaving as both despicable and sinful.

"I had grown a splendid moustache, which was the envy of all the boys abroad, and which all the advice of Drs Ogle and Greenhill failed to make me remove. I declined to be shaved until formal orders were issued by the authorities of the college. For I had already formed strong ideas upon the Shaven Age of England."
—Sir Richard Burton (1821–90)

For a time, British trends and innovations in both facial hairstyles and shaving predominated, but by 1880, Americans started to lead the race. That year, the Kampfe brothers patented a safety razor which incorporated a wire guard along one edge of the razor to protect the skin. Fifteen years later, Baltimore salesman King Camp Gillette decided that he was destined to strike it rich by marketing something disposable but absolutely indispensable. In 1895, he dreamed up a disposable razor blade, an idea he acquired from a friend of his who had invented throwaway bottle caps. However, no technology for its manufacture would exist until 1901, when he hooked up with William Nickerson, an MIT engineer (and inventor of several wonders, including the push-button for elevators).

They improved on the safety razor by producing a double-edge blade cut from a template, which could be dropped onto the top of a T-shaped razor, then used, discarded, and more importantly, replaced over and over. In 1903, they went into production—and a whopping fifty razors were sold. But by 1906, 300,000 razors and 500,000 blades were purchased. A UK office soon opened.

When World War I began, the US government ordered 3.5 million razors and 36 million blades for its soldiers. By the 1920s, a safety razor designed for women appeared, women having been convinced that underarm hair was nasty and unfeminine. Alas, the ubiquity of razors helped cut down the Victorian mustache movement in its prime!

The *schnurbartbinde* was a German mustache trainer used in the early 1900s.

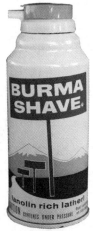

And what of other shaving staples we take for granted today, like the electric razor or fancy foams? In 1906, W.G. Shockey patented the first wind-up safety razor, which became extremely popular until supplanted twenty years later by the plug-in. In 1925, a brushless, convenient-to-use shaving cream called Burma Shave came out of Minneapolis, Minnesota, reportedly derived from a native recipe picked up by sailors stationed in Burma. By 1936, it became a top seller and grew in popularity because of an ingenious campaign using hundreds of billboards with

1960s Burma Shave can. Photo, Roadsidepictures, 2006.

clever slogans mounted along particularly boring strips of US highway. Sadly, this icon of both shaving and advertising stopped production in 1966, until it was reintroduced by the American Safety Razor Company in 1997.

The next big name in shaving was Jacob Schick, who was single-handedly responsible for the distinction between a "wet" shave (i.e., razor) and a "dry" shave (i.e., electric), improving significantly on both. He invented and, by 1926, marketed a magazine-repeating razor which housed twenty spare blades in its razor handle, advanced with a plunger. The consumer didn't have to touch them and could buy clips of blades as replacements. Schick was also a US lieutenant colonel, and while stationed in some godforsaken, cold country, he injured his ankle and had to crawl out of bed to crack, then melt, ice in order to shave (a story that sounds a bit embellished to me); like all inventors, he told himself that there "had to be a better way." Sure enough, by 1927 he invented the first electric shaver, which used oscillating blades, and two years later he began to sell them. The unit was initially unwieldy because of a cumbersome motor, but by 1931, Schick sold 3,000 at the unthinkable price of twenty-five dollars each.

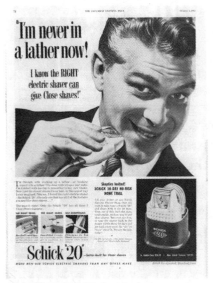

Ad for the Schick 20 electric shaver. *Saturday Evening Post*, Oct. 3, 1953.

Shockey's wind-up razor continued to give him a run for

his money until electric dry shaving caught on, especially with travelers. By the 1930s, most airplanes, ships, and trains had outlets for electric shavers, something we observe to this day. (I confess I have never dared use one, fearing a jolt from the engine or a thrust into the mirror.) Imitators quickly followed. In 1936, Sunbeam introduced the Shavemaster. Remington launched the Close Shaver in 1937, the same year the ingenious Colonel Schick died in Canada. It was clear that as long as men eschewed the beard, technocrats would be at the drawing board whipping up some pricey new twist on shaving.

In 1939, Philips, the company founded by Dutchman Gerard Philips and his father Frederik, began to market an electric razor that had two heads and a rotary blade. By the late 1940s, a battery-powered shaver, which freed men from wall outlets, appeared on the market. Electric razors became part of the masculine cultural landscape, suggesting both affluence and modernity. Many popular films from that era have scenes of prominent actors shaving with dry razors; Jimmy Stewart uses one in *Rear Window* (1954), as does Humphrey Bogart in *Sabrina* (also 1954). In 1960, Remington introduced the rechargeable shaver and Philips announced a triple header in 1966. By 1969, one-third of men in the UK and two-thirds in the US were using electric razors. In 1978, Victor Kiam famously "liked [his] Remington razor so much that [he] bought the company." Until his death in 2001, his television ads proved to be

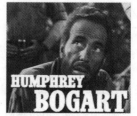

Humphrey Bogart in a screenshot from the trailer for the film *The Treasure of the Sierra Madre*, 1948.

as annoying as they were ubiquitous and effective. By 1981, Philips and its US branch, Norelco, took over Schick's products and trademarks. All the while, electric shaving machines grew more sleek, "masculine," and ultra-modern with elaborate leather (or leatherette) travel cases, suggesting jet-setting savoir-faire.

But while converts flocked to dry shaving, the wet shave industry would not be outdone. The race for sleek product design and "close, closer, closest" was on. Oregon lumberjacks may still have been shaving with axes in the 1930s, but an entire industry sought to convince men that a wholesome, clean shave could only be achieved by a blade. The Gem Cutlery Company, with its "Gem" razor, cleverly coined the phrase "five o' clock shadow" to describe and discourage midday break-through stubble. Aftershaves—cosmetic toners and moisturizers, though God forbid they should be called that—started to appear; they were virile-sounding products

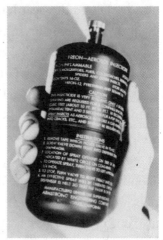

Aerosol spray canister invented by USDA researchers, 1943.

with associated macho mythologies: Aqua Velva in 1935; Old Spice in 1938; English Leather in 1949; and Brut in 1964. Aerosol foam appeared in cans in 1949, replacing shaving soap, mugs, and brushes. Pinaud-Clubman has long supplied mustache wax for stache twirlers; dozens of new mustache-wax companies have sprung up in the last ten years, reflecting the big-time return of the mo.

**In 1969, a Chicago group called Mustache Growers Ltd. declared the day after Labor Day to be Natural Mustache Day, "a day of recognition for mustache cultivators." This was the first official call for a widespread, ongoing celebration of the mo.
—*The Milwaukee Journal,* September 2, 1975.**

Naturally, a market split of the adult population between "wet" and "dry" continued to stimulate fierce competitions and industrial innovation. Gillette marketed "long lasting" stainless steel blades in 1960. Though available as early as 1945, cartridge razors reappeared and were heavily marketed through the take-out, throwaway '60s and '70s. (No one worried about landfills back then.) The most popular of these were produced by Frenchman Marcel Bich (of "Flick Your Bic" fame), who introduced his yellow disposables in 1972. A design war proliferated: razors needed to be even more high-tech, scientific, reliable, sharp, and earnest, like the men who used them. If shaving was an unconscious act of castration, then the man performing it needed a state-of-the-art tool that rendered him macho and restored his sense of self.

In 1971, Gillette marketed a twin-bladed razor called the Trac 2. Six years later, it introduced a pivoting head which followed the contours of the face, called Atra (automatic tracking razor), an acronym suggesting a space-age defence program.

By the 1990s, "comfort strips" were available, containing lubricants or polyvinyl above the blades. The new "sensitive" male of the '90s wasn't afraid to cry and didn't seem to mind being told that he also had sensitive skin. In 1998, Mach 3, a triple-bladed razor, was launched by Gillette after top-secret research that allegedly cost the company almost $750 million. Interestingly, the advertising budget for all razors seems to have dropped in the 1980s, but has exploded of late; the razor companies are now busily investing their money in the next new gizmo, which they will soon convince us will revolutionize shaving yet again.

According to a survey of New York City barbers, requests for stache trims increased by a third in 2010.

And what will that look like? We're up to quintuple razors and electric shavers that you can use wet or dry. And whatever the latest facial-hair craze will be, shaving companies will follow them closely; it didn't take them long to unleash a new batch of high-tech electric clippers for ultra-precise goatee pruning, sideburn trimming, stache clipping, and soul patch shaping. Stubble has been a very popular look in recent years—a look that requires precise electric upkeep—worn alongside a full stache. It is clear that no matter what tools are available, fashion trends and perceptions of masculine power will continue to dictate whether a man shaves or grows. I would argue that the modern fellow with a mustache has the best of both worlds—the opportunity to both shave and grow!

How Many Ways Can You Say "Mustache"?
British author Adam Jacot de Boinod has claimed
that the Albanian language has twenty-seven
words for the mustache. Ironically wearing one
(wearing any kind of facial hair, in fact) was
banned in Albania in the mid-1970s under the rule
of Albanian dictator Enver Hoxha, who felt they
were unhygienic, and who also wanted to restrain
the rights of bearded Muslims and the Orthodox.

In 2012 the American Mustache Institute (cheekily) called for a $250 tax credit for the cost of grooming supplies required, i.e., stache upkeep.

THE RELIGIOUS MO

Throughout history, beards, mustaches, and other forms of facial hair have always been important, easily visible signs of belonging (or excommunication) within religious communities. Muslims, Sikhs, Jews, and various sects of Christians have strong opinions about facial hair and what it means to cut it, shape it, or remove it. Often, it is suggested that those who choose to shave are spiritually misguided or worse, "infidels."

Mohammad (570–632 CE) instructed his followers to trim their mustaches and to allow their beards to grow. (The beard was defined as hair on the cheeks and jaws, and also included the temples and growth under the lower lip, chin, and sideburns.) Mohammad specified that the mustache be clipped so as not to enter the mouth. It is believed that he insisted on this to distinguish Muslims from Christians and from the long-mustachioed Zoroastrians. Growing a beard and mustache, in Islam, is thus mandatory for all men capable of doing so. It represents some of the qualities for a good and clean nature prized by Muslims. Sunni Muslims, however, may shave their staches.

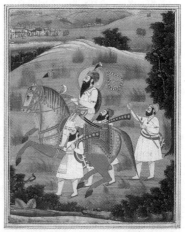

Guru Gobind Singh, ca. 1830.

For Sikhs, the followers of Gobind Singh (1666–1708), five symbols signify the Khalsa, or tenets of the faith. These are commonly known as the Five Ks and included Kes or Kesh, which stipulates the wearing of uncut hair with an unshaven beard and mustache (but never a stache alone).

In fact, in most religions, the mustache was seldom worn alone. For Jews, instructions on the wearing of beards can be found in Leviticus 19:27: "Ye shall not round the corners of your heads, neither shalt thou mar the corners of thy beard." The Jews also used their facial hair to distinguish themselves from their enemies at the time, including the Romans, Egyptians, and early Christians.

Things were a little less clear for those early Christians. Although the Old Testament abounds with references to the beard and mustache, the New Testament is strangely silent on the subject, even though Christ himself wore a beard like his contemporaries. This surprising absence of commentary has allowed theologians and clergymen throughout the ages to conclude that Christian men were either obliged to shave, grow beards, or defer the decision altogether. Christian religious communities throughout history either forbade the beard, encouraged its growth, or taxed it. At various points, the mustache was considered to be the mark of the Beast, as

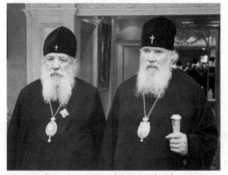

it was thought to interfere with receiving communion or holy wine from the chalice. In 1587, for example, religious councils ordered that the mo be "kept clear of the upper lip." Orthodox Christian clergy let the beard and stache grow in emula-

Metropolitan Laurus and Patriarch Alexius in Moscow. И. Максим photo, 2008.

tion of the monastic ascetics of the desert—and to distinguish themselves from their clean-shaven Roman Catholic counterparts.

For Amish and Hutterite men, untrimmed beards indicate marital status, but they are not allowed to grow mustaches, which are associated with the military. Their pacifism is thus symbolized by a bare upper lip.

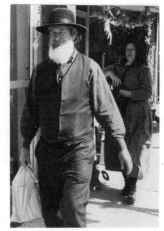

Amish couple shopping in Aylmer, Ontario, Canada.

While the mustache has been popular among Indian men, neither Hindu nor Buddhist doctrines set out rules or instructions regarding its growth or maintenance; in India, the mustache thus may be more of a patriarchal than strictly religious symbol. Young, hip Buddhists, however, are quick to point out that the young Buddha, i.e., Prince Siddhartha, is often portrayed wearing a mustache.

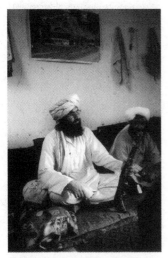

Taliban border guard in Torkham, Afghanistan, 2001.

Under the Taliban, Afghani men were obliged to grow beards at least four inches long, a sort of hairy veil marking obedience.

"Looking for peace is like looking for a turtle with a mustache: You won't be able to find it. But when your heart is ready, peace will come looking for you."
—Venerable Ajahn Chah, Buddhist teacher

THE POLITICAL MO

Over the centuries and in various countries, facial hair has symbolized a range of political affiliations, from right-wing to radical left, and it's also signified anti-establishment protest. Staches have both bolstered and weakened the political careers of their wearers, depending on the tenor of the times. In modern-day Turkey, the size and shape of a mustache indicates its wearer's political views. If the mo is full with down-turned ends at the corners of the mouth, it likely belongs to a right-wing nationalist. If it's a small brush stache, it's likely being worn by a follower of political Islam. A long mustache drooping over the upper lip is a sign of being an old-fashioned leftist.

Certain cultural communities, such as African Americans in the United States, have always embraced the mustache—and not as a fashion or fad. It can be argued that the stache has been a powerful symbol of their racial difference from the clean-shaven white majority and emblematic of community-building and cultural survival. (Think of the staches of Martin Luther King, Jr. and Jessie Jackson.)

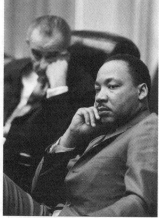

President Lyndon B. Johnson and Rev. Dr. Martin Luther King, Jr. meet at the White House, 1966.

On the other hand, the last British prime minister to wear a mustache was Harold Macmillan (1894–1986). It has been argued (most notably by Piers Brendon in *The Decline and Fall of the British Empire*) that Macmillan's mustache became a symbol of England's waning influence as the empire faded.

Mid-century US politics affords us another example of the sometimes deleterious effect of the mo: Thomas E. Dewey (1902–71) was a young stache-sporting lawyer (his nickname was "the Mustache") and rising Republican. It's been

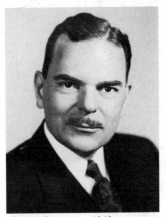

suggested that Dewey's mo may have ended his political career. Christopher Oldstone-Moore, in an article about the "performative function of facial hair" published in the *Journal of Social History*, has suggested that by the 1940s the stache was a political liability because it indicated that the wearer was not a team player, but prone to being unpredictable and willfully inde-

Thomas Dewey ca. 1948.

pendent. In 1948, Dewey won the Republican presidential nomination, and most pollsters and the press predicted that he would win the presidency itself—but he lost by a, well, a hair. (There is a famous photo of his successful opponent, clean-shaven Democrat Harry S. Truman, holding up a newspaper with the headline, "Dewey Defeats Truman.")

A DOZEN POLITICO MUSTACHES

These politicians and statesmen have lent gravitas to a furry lip and have steadfastly done the mo proud:

- Kofi Annan: Seventh Secretary-General of the United Nations, 1997–2006
- Chester A. Arthur: US President, 1881–85
- Neville Chamberlain: Prime Minister of the United Kingdom, 1937–40

- Grover Cleveland: US President, 1885–89 and 1893–97

- Vicente Fox: President of Mexico, 2000–2006

- Mohandas Karamchand Gandhi: leader of the Indian Independence movement

- Martin Luther King, Jr.: clergyman and leader of the African-American Civil Rights Movement

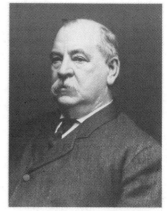

Grover Cleveland.

- Harold Macmillan: Prime Minister of the United Kingdom, 1957–63

- Theodore "Teddy" Roosevelt: US President, 1901–09

- Anwar Sadat: Third President of Egypt

- William Howard Taft: US President, 1909–13

- Lech Wałęsa: President of Poland, 1990–95, and Solidarity trade union co-founder

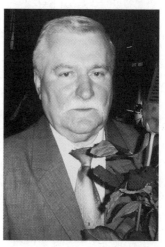

Lech Wałęsa, 2007.

Nobel Peace Prize-winning, freedom-fighting, mo-wearing Lech Wałęsa, who once insisted he was born with a mustache, shaved his off in 2002 and refused to explain why.

THE NATIONALIST STACHE

The following countries have long been, and continue to be, stache friendly. Mustaches can be seen on the streets of these places, but are also worn by the men who emmigrated to others parts of the world carrying their proud stache traditions with them. The American Mustache Institute listed these countries in 2011:

1. Bulgaria: perhaps as a remote reference to Turkish occupation

2. Egypt: where presidents Gamal Abdel Nasser and Anwar Sadat both had excellent mustaches

3. Germany: the land of Bismarck, Nietzsche, Einstein, and the first World Beard and Moustache Championship

4. Hungary: where a fine Magyar military-stache tradition has existed for more than 1,000 years

5. India: where eighty percent of the men in the south wear staches

6. Iran: a throwback to those fine Persian mo's

7. Mexico: in honor of Mexican Revolutionary leader Emiliano Zapata

8. Pakistan: where philosopher-poet Mohammed Iqbal and former president Pervez Musharraf both wore mo's

9. Turkey: where the bulk, twirl, and point of your stache indicate your political allegiance

10. United States: where the most mustache-friendly cities are said to be Chicago, Houston, Pittsburg, Oklahoma City, Detroit, Milwaukee, Cleveland, New York, Huntsville, and Tampa-St. Petersburg-Clearwater

Poland has embraced the mustache since the days of Jan Sobieski, the country's king from 1674 to 1696. His handlebar was copied by aristocrats and commoners alike; the style has never really gone away and has become an enduring emblem of patriotism. Later, poet Franciszek Dionizy Kniaźnin mocked the French fashion of shaving in a number of his poems. Joseph Conrad, the Polish-born novelist, made sure a number of his characters had mo's.

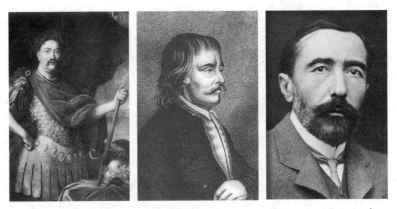

Jerzy Szymonowicz, *Portrait of John III Sobieski*, ca. 1693, oil on canvas, Franciszek Dionizy Kniaźnin, late 18th c., Joseph Conrad, 1904.

The Moustache Brothers are a group of comedic satirists in Burma. Two of the troupe's members are mo-wearing brothers who have satirized the oppressive regime in their country, surviving sanction and imprisonment, but just by a hair.

Policemen in large Indian cities are sometimes paid a bonus if they grow a mustache because it is considered a symbol of virility and power.

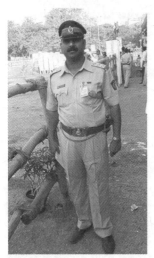

An Indian police inspector during Republic Day Parade, Mumbai, 2009.

Canada's most famous mustachioed leader was Robert Borden, prime minister from 1911 to 1920.

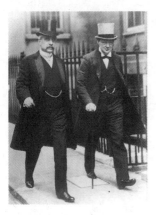

Canadian Prime Minister Robert Borden (1854–1937) and Winston Churchill (then First Lord of the Admiralty) in 1912.

MUSTACHE TYRANTS IN HISTORY

The mustache has come to be associated with evil, war-mongering, and cultural genocide. Blame this horrible lot for many of the negative historical and cultural associations we have about the mo:

- Genghis Khan (1162–1227): Mongolian warlord and famous conqueror

- Gilles de Montmorency-Laval, Baron de Rais (1404–40): Breton knight and serial child-killer

- Vlad the Impaler (1431–76): Prince of Wallachia, otherwise known as Count Dracula

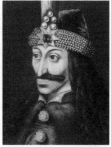

- Tala'at Pasha (1847–1921): ordered the genocide of the Ottoman Empire's Armenian population

- Kaiser Wilhelm II (1859–1941): last German Emperor and King of Prussia who supported Austria-Hungary in the crisis of 1914, leading to World War I

Vlad Tepes (Vlad the Impaler), 16th c.

- Joseph Stalin (1879–1953): Soviet dictator under whose regime millions of people were killed

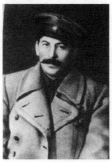

- Adolf Hitler (1889–1945): Der Führer's "New Order" called for the extinction of Jews, gays, gypsies, and the mentally and physically disabled

- Francisco Franco (1892–1975): Spanish military dictator who overthrew a democratically elected government in the Spanish Civil War

Joseph Stalin, 1919.

- Heinrich Himmler (1900–21): Reichsführer of the Nazi SS and overseer of their concentration camps

- Hirohito, Emperor Showa (1901–89): Emperor of Japan; invaded China in 1937 and attacked the US in the Pacific Ocean during World War II

- Augusto Pinochet (1915–2006): Chilean army general and dictator who "disappeared" thousands of Chilean citizens during his reign of terror

- Robert Mugabe (1924–): controversial and tyrannical President of Zimbabwe

- Saddam Hussein (1937–2006): repressive dictator of Iraq until his overthrow in a US-led invasion in 2003

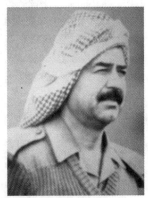

Saddam Hussein, 1982.

Saddam Hussein kept a retinue of mustachioed imposters to mislead those making attempts on his life. Hussein insisted that all his senior officials wear his trademark Ba'athist mo. He reputedly said, "A man who holds his mustache holds his honor." Not surprisingly, many Iraqi men took up the razor after his capture.

Hitler's Mustache Myth: It's been said that Hitler chopped his previously pointed Prussian stache in order to fit into a gas mask. In fact, the toothbrush stache was popular in the German military, but after World War II, the style became practically taboo.

MO PHOBIA AND PROTEST

Men of the stache have never taken things lying down. Here's what's happened in the past when their mo's were threatened:

In 1907, Parisian waiters marched through the streets when their trademark staches were forbidden by an ill-conceived ordinance. European waiters have always been champions of the stache.

In July 1966, the new military regime in Argentina closed the satirical magazine Tia Vicenta, partly for referring to generalisi-mo Juan Carlos Onganía as a "walrus." Ironically, that nickname had been popularized by his colleagues in the Argentine Armed Forces.

In November 1966, 350 college students in Grand Rapids, Michigan, walked out of class to protest a ban on mo's on campus.

In March 2000, a longstanding stache ban for Disney theme-park employees was lifted. (Walt Disney had a stache himself.) In January 2012, employees were finally allowed to wear beards.

In 2007, **workers** at the Terrapin Beer Company in Georgia grew mustaches in protest over a delay in the issue of a state brewing license.

In 2008, **a group** of French feminists wearing fake fuzz and calling themselves La Barbe (which means "the beard," and is also used idiomatically to mean "enough") and their counterparts from Mexico, Las Bigotinas ("the mustached ones"), staged high-profile protests at cultural and political events to protest sexism in the media.

In **July 2009**, Brazilian men staged a greve de bigode (mustache strike) as a protest against political corruption perpetrated by the president of the senate, Jose Sarney de Araujo Costa (who had a bushy stache himself).

THE MILITARY MO

We've seen how, early in human history, the mustache became a powerful symbol of military might, starting with the barbarian tribes and sweeping across Europe. Most countries in Europe and America today allow their soldiers to wear well-kept, trimmed mustaches, although many have prohibited full beards because they interfere with proper seals on safety masks. Norway and Finland, however, have banned all mustaches as well as beards.

In the Canadian army, "mustaches are permitted provided they are neatly trimmed and do not extend beyond the corners of the mouth. The handlebar mustache, however, is permitted. In no case is a beard permitted without a mustache."

FRANCE

Ever since Napoleonic times and throughout the nineteenth century, the French army wore beards; however, the Grenadiers, which were elite troops, wore large mustaches. Infantrymen wore smaller mustaches, sometimes with goatees. Many of these facial hair traditions were discontinued in the twentieth century, except for men in the French Foreign Legion, who to this day are encouraged to grow large beards. The mustache was obligatory for French *gendarmes* (policemen) until 1933, and many still carry on that fine tradition.

BRITAIN

The United Kingdom has a glorious facial hair and mustache tradition, which as we've seen emerged in the early nineteenthcentury when the British mustache was inspired by two foreign influences. The Napoleonic War (1792–1815) saw British officers emulating their French counterparts, whose mustaches were said to be "appurtenances of terror." In India, the Brits started to adapt the customs of the locals, who viewed the clean-shaven English face as unmanly. The British colonial rulers wore mustaches to appear daunting, aggressive, and in control. Nonetheless, Lord Dalhousie (1812–60), the Governor General of India, criticized what he called the "capillary decorations" of his officers. But by 1854, they were made mandatory for the troops of the East India Company's Bombay Army.

During the Crimean War, English barbers offered special services for the mustache. They could be clipped, trimmed, pointed, curved, waxed, and made erect. The foot guards were the first to allow all ranks to grow large mustaches during the Crimean War, and the trend spread to other parts of the British military.

From the late 1800s until 1916, British soldiers were forbidden to shave their upper lips. But that regulation was abolished on October 6, 1916 by Lieutenant-General Sir Nevil Macready, who apparently detested having to

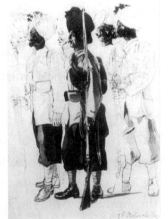

AC Lovett, *30th Regiment Bombay Infantry*, 1890, charcoal and watercolor.

wear a mustache and shaved his own off immediately. Since then, the Royal Navy has allowed a full set, i.e., a beard and a mustache, but not beards or mustaches alone. While the army, air force, and marines allow mustaches, their men may still be able to grow full beards if they have documented religious or medical exemptions. Two styles of mustaches are still permitted in the British army: a neatly trimmed mustache that does not extend beyond the corners of the upper lip or over its upper edge, or a waxed handlebar mustache, provided it does not extend beyond the corners of the mouth and angles neatly upward. Its length must not exceed the uppermost point of growth below the nostrils.

Overall, the demise of the British mustache seems to have gone hand-in-hand with the demise of the British empire, as the twentieth century progressed.

"She had much in common with Hitler, only no moustache." —Noel Coward, speaking of Mary Baker Eddy, the founder of Christian Science

THE UNITED STATES

While all branches of the US military currently prohibit beards, mustaches are still allowed, based on rules that were established during World War I. According to Section 2, Article 2201.2, which details Grooming Standards for the US Navy, mustaches "should be kept neatly and closely trimmed. No portion of the mustache shall extend below the lip line of the upper lip. It shall not go beyond the horizontal line extending across the corners of the mouth, and no more than one-quarter inch beyond a vertical line drawn from the corner of the mouth. The length of an individual mustache hair fully extended should not extend approximately one-half inch (Fig. 2.2.1). Handlebar mustaches, goatees, beards or eccentricities are not permitted."

In the marine corps, "the face will be clean shaven, except that a mustache may be worn. When worn, a mustache will be neatly trimmed and must be contained within imaginary vertical lines from the corners of the mouth and the imaginary line of the upper lip. The individual length of a mustache hair fully extended must not exceed one-half inch."

In the air force, mustaches may not extend "beyond the lip line of the upper lip or sideways beyond a vertical line drawn upward from the corners of the mouth."

Ouch!: In the Napoleonic era, European military officers were said to shape their military mo's with hot tar. Talk about a stiff upper lip!

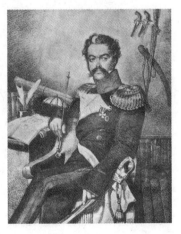

Portrait of Denis Davydov (1784–1839), a Russian soldier-poet of the Napoleonic Wars.

In March 1918, the US War Department agreed to pay for a shaving kit for every enlisted soldier.

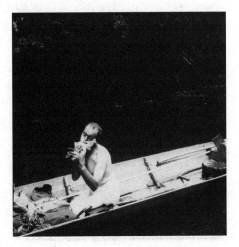

Military in a canoe while shaving, 1948, Tropenmuseum of the Royal Tropical Institute (KIT) Collection.

Many a thief has donned a fake stache, believing it was an instant disguise. One famous heist was perpetrated in Boston in 1990 by men dressed as cops with staches. They got away with $500,000 worth of paintings by Rembrandt, Vermeer, Degas, and Manet.

THE LITERARY AND ARTISTIC MO

Writers, painters, and musicians have long been associated with the bohemian lifestyle, and our image of the struggling, romantic artist comes to us from the nineteenth century, when the mo was in full swing. In garrets and galleries, concert halls and publishing houses throughout Europe and North America, artists with an assortment of mo styles were everywhere to be seen. Edgar Allan Poe wore a well-trimmed Chevron mustache while writing his macabre stories and poems. The creator of Sherlock Holmes, Sir Arthur Conan

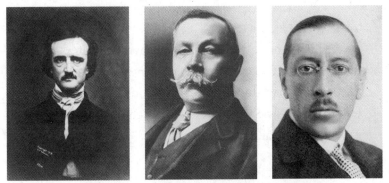

Edgar Allan Poe, 1848, Arthur Conan Doyle, 1914, and Igor Stravinsky, 1921.

Doyle, waxed the inch-long tips of his handlebar so that they stood out stiffly to the sides. Composer Maurice Ravel was painted by Impressionist artist Henri Charles Manquin wearing what we would now call a "Zappa" mustache. Russian composer Igor Stravinksy had a modest Pyramid stache under his large nose, while French composer Gabriel Fauré sported an enormous Walrus.

However, lest you think that the great artists of earlier eras didn't stroke their whiskers in thoughtful moments of inspired creativity, have a look at the upper lips of both William Shakespeare and Geoffrey Chaucer, both of whom sported staches paired with natty goatees.

"The moustaches are glorious, glorious. I have cut them shorter and trimmed them a little at the ends to improve their shape. They are charming. Without them, life would be a blank."
—Charles Dickens

THE WRITE STACHE

If you think about it, many of your favorite writers probably had mo's. Particularly in the nineteenth and early twentieth centuries, the mustache was often associated with spectacular literary prowess. See how you do matching these ink-stached men to one of their famous works:

1. William Shakespeare (ca. 1564–1616)

2. Edgar Allan Poe (1809–1849)

3. Gustave Flaubert (1821–1880)

4. Mark Twain (1835–1910)

5. Guy de Maupassant (1850–1893)

6. Arthur Conan Doyle (1859–1930)

7. Rudyard Kipling (1865–1936)

8. W. Somerset Maugham (1874–1965)

9. E.M. Forster
   (1879–1970)

10. James Joyce
    (1882–1941)

11. William Faulkner
    (1897–1962)

12. Ernest Hemingway
    (1899–1961)

13. George Orwell
    (1903–1950)

14. Tennessee Williams
    (1911–1983)

15. Gabriel García
    Márquez (1928–)

16. Edward Albee (1928–)

17. John Barth (1930–)

18. Salman Rushdie
    (1947–)

A. *A Streetcar Named Desire*

B. *Animal Farm*

C. *For Whom the Bell Tolls*

D. *Giles Goat-Boy*

E. *Madame Bovary*

F. *Maurice*

G. "Mother Savage"

H. *Of Human Bondage*

I. *One Hundred Years of Solitude*

J. *The Adventures of Sherlock Holmes*

K. *The Adventures of Tom Sawyer*

L. *The Jungle Book*

M. "The Raven"

N. *The Satanic Verses*

O. *The Sound and the Fury*

P. *The Tempest*

Q. *Ulysses*

R. *Who's Afraid of Virginia Woolf?*

Answers: 1-P; 2-M; 3-E; 4-K; 5-G; 6-J; 7-L; 8-H; 9-F; 10-Q; 11-O; 12-C; 13-B; 14-A; 15-I; 16-R; 17-D; 18-N

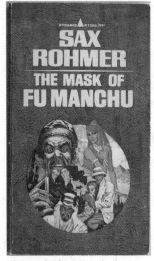

Fu Manchu was the name of a diabolical villain created by novelist Sax Rohmer. The character actually had no mo in the novels, but was given the style we know and love in Hollywood adaptations of the books.

The Mask of Fu Manchu by Sax Rohmer Book cover photo, Chris Drumm.

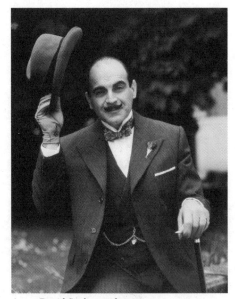

Agatha Christie announced the death of Hercule Poirot, her beloved Belgian detective with the iconic stache, in 1975.

Actor David Suchet as detective Hercule Poirot, 1988.

"THERE IS NO LOVE WITHOUT A MUSTACHE!"

"The Mustache," by Guy de Maupassant (1850–93), mustachioed short story writer, tells the tale of a wife whose husband shaves his stache for a theatrical role. In this epistolic tale, she melodramatically laments its disappearance in a letter to a friend:

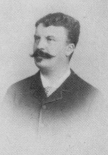

Guy de Maupassant
(1850–1893)

Chateau De Solles, July 30, 1883

My Dear Lucy,

I have no news. We live in the drawing-room, looking out at the rain. We cannot go out in this frightful weather, so we have theatricals. How stupid they are, my dear, these drawing entertainments in the repertory of real life! All is forced, coarse, heavy. The jokes are like cannon balls, smashing everything in their passage. No wit, nothing natural, no sprightliness, no elegance. These literary men, in truth, know nothing of society. They are perfectly ignorant of how people think and talk in our set. I do not mind if they despise our customs, our conventionalities, but I do not forgive them for not knowing them. When they want to be humorous they make puns that would do for a barrack; when they try to be jolly, they give us jokes that they must have picked up on the outer boulevard in those beer houses artists are supposed to frequent, where one has heard the same students' jokes for fifty years.

So we have taken to Theatricals. As we are only two women, my husband takes the part of a soubrette, and, in order to do that, he has shaved off his mustache. You cannot imagine, my dear Lucy, how it changes him! I no longer recognize him—by day or at night. If he did not let it grow again I think I should no longer love him;

he looks so horrid like this.

In fact, a man without a mustache is no longer a man. I do not care much for a beard; it almost always makes a man look untidy. But a mustache, oh, a mustache is indispensable to a manly face. No, you would never believe how these little hair bristles on the upper lip are a relief to the eye and good in other ways. I have thought over the matter a great deal but hardly dare to write my thoughts. Words look so different on paper and the subject is so difficult, so delicate, so dangerous that it requires infinite skill to tackle it.

Well, when my husband appeared, shaven, I understood at once that I never could fall in love with a strolling actor nor a preacher, even if it were Father Didon, the most charming of all! Later when I was alone with him (my husband) it was worse still. Oh, my dear Lucy, never let yourself be kissed by a man without a mustache; their kisses have no flavor, none whatever! They no longer have the charm, the mellowness and the snap—yes, the snap—of a real kiss. The mustache is the spice.

Imagine placing to your lips a piece of dry—or moist— parchment. That is the kiss of the man without a mustache. It is not worthwhile.

Whence comes this charm of the mustache, will you tell me? Do I know myself? It tickles your face, you feel it approaching your mouth and it sends a little shiver through you down to the tips of your toes.

And on your neck! Have you ever felt a mustache on your neck? It intoxicates you, makes you feel creepy, goes to the tips of your fingers. You wriggle, shake your shoulders, toss back your head. You wish to get away and at the same time to remain there; it is delightful, but irritating. But how good it is!

A lip without a mustache is like a body without clothing; and one must wear clothes, very few, if you like, but still some clothing.

I recall a sentence (uttered by a politician) which has been running in my mind for three months. My husband, who keeps up with the newspapers, read me one evening a very singular speech by our Minister of Agriculture, who was called M. Meline. He may have been superseded by this time. I do not know.

I was paying no attention, but the name Meline struck me. It recalled, I do not exactly know why, the "Scenes de la vie de boheme." I thought it was about some grisette. That shows how scraps of the speech entered my mind. This M. Meline was making this statement to the people of Amiens, I believe, and I have ever since been trying to understand what he meant: "There is no patriotism without agriculture!" Well, I have just discovered his meaning, and I affirm in my turn that there is no love without a mustache. When you say it that way it sounds comical, does it not?

There is no love without a mustache!

"There is no patriotism without agriculture," said M. Meline, and he was right, that minister; I now understand why.

From a very different point of view the mustache is essential. It gives character to the face. It makes a man look gentle, tender, violent, a monster, a rake, enterprising! The hairy man, who does not shave off his whiskers, never has a refined look, for his features are concealed; and the shape of the jaw and the chin betrays a great deal to those who understand.

The man with a mustache retains his own peculiar expression and his refinement at the same time.

And how many different varieties of mustaches there are! Sometimes they are twisted, curled, coquettish. Those seem to be chiefly devoted to women.

Sometimes they are pointed, sharp as needles, and threatening.

That kind prefers wine, horses and war.

Sometimes they are enormous, overhanging, frightful. These big ones generally conceal a fine disposition, a kindliness that borders on weakness and a gentleness that savors of timidity.

But what I adore above all in the mustache is that it is French, altogether French. It came from our ancestors, the Gauls, and has remained the insignia of our national character.

It is boastful, gallant and brave. It sips wine gracefully and knows how to laugh with refinement, while the broad-bearded jaws are clumsy in everything they do.

I recall something that made me weep all my tears and also—I see it now—made me love a mustache on a man's face. It was during the war, when I was living with my father. I was a young girl then. One day there was a skirmish near the chateau. I had heard the firing of the cannon and of the artillery all the morning, and that evening a German colonel came and took up his abode in our house. He left the following day.

My father was informed that there were a number of dead bodies in the fields. He had them brought to our place so that they might be buried together. They were laid all along the great avenue of pines as fast as they brought them in, on both sides of the avenue, and as they began to smell unpleasant, their bodies were covered with earth until the deep trench could be dug. Thus one saw only their heads which seemed to protrude from the clayey earth and were almost as yellow, with their closed eyes.

I wanted to see them. But when I saw those two rows of frightful faces, I thought I should faint. However, I began to look at them, one by one, trying to guess what kind of men these had been.

The uniforms were concealed beneath the earth, and yet immediately, yes, immediately, my dear, I recognized the Frenchmen by their mustache!

Some of them had shaved on the very day of the battle, as though they wished to be elegant up to the last; others seemed to have a week's growth, but all wore the French mustache, very plain, the proud mustache that seems to say: Do not take me for my bearded friend, little one; I am a brother."

And I cried, oh, I cried a great deal more than I should if I had not recognized them, the poor dead fellows.

It was wrong of me to tell you this. Now I am sad and cannot chatter any longer. Well, good-bye, dear Lucy. I send you a hearty kiss. Long live the mustache!

Jeanne

THE ART OF THE MO

No discussion on the artistic or creative mustache can be complete without paying tribute to an iconic mo-mater and mo-pater: two brilliant painters whose staches are arguably as well-known as their impressive bodies of work.

FRIDA KAHLO (1907–54)

This Mexican painter repeatedly painted herself stache and all because, as she said, "I am so often alone and because I am the subject I know best." While her female contemporaries spent millions to eradicate unwanted facial hair, Kahlo's became an emblem of her Latin American pride, bisexuality, androgyny, communism, rebellion, and indefatigable will in the face of chronic physical suffering caused by an accident she suffered as a young woman.

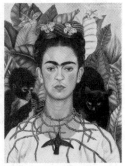

Frida Kahlo, *Self-Portrait with Thorn Necklace and Hummingbird*, 1940, oil on canvas.

SALVADOR DALI (1904–89)

This Catalan-Spanish Surrealist painter was rumored (apocryphally) to use his stache as a brush when he couldn't afford art supplies. Photographs of Dali regularly showed him with his outrageous stache waxed so that it extended several inches from his face. In 1954, with photographer Philippe Halsman, Dali wrote a tribute to his impossibly expressive mo. called *Dali's Mustache*: "With the points of its hair, I can paint a fly with all the details of his hair. And while I am painting my fly, I think philosophically of my mustache, to which all the flies and all the curiosities of my era came to be monotonously and irresistibly stuck. Someday perhaps we will discover a truth almost as strange as this mustache—namely, that Salvador Dali was possibly also a painter." (Philippe Halsman, *Dali's Mustache: A Photographic Interview.*)

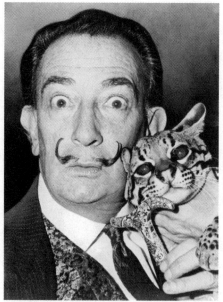

"Since I don't smoke, I decided to grow a mustache—it is better for the health."
—Salvador Dali

Salvador Dali with ocelot and cane, 1965.

Another Famous Lady with a Stache: Simone "Eleanor Dumont" Jules, a.k.a. Madame Mustache, was an infamous Wild West scam-gambler who cleaned out the poker winnings of many a Gold Rush prospector in the 1850s.

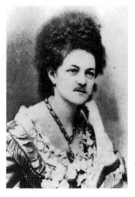

THE CLASSIC(AL) STACHE

These composers, all contemporaries of one another, may owe much to their lyrical mo's:

- Alexander Borodin (1833–1887): Russian Romantic
- Anton Bruckner (1824–1896): Austrian master of dissonance
- Paul Dukas (1865–1935): Frenchman best known for *The Sorcerer's Apprentice*
- Antonín Dvořák (1841–1904): Czech composer of late Romantic works
- Edward Elgar (1857–1934): Englishman who knew about *Pomp and Circumstance*
- Gabriel Fauré (1845–1924): French composer of "Clair de lune"
- Edvard Grieg (1843–1907): Norwegian composer of piano miniatures
- Giacomo Puccini (1858–1924): Italian creator of *Madama Butterfly*

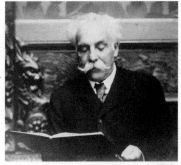

Gabriel Fauré, 1907.

- Maurice Ravel (1875–1937): French composer of *Boléro*

- Igor Stravinsky (1882–1971): Russian composer of *The Rite of Spring*

- Karol Szymanowski (1882–1937): Polish composer and pianist

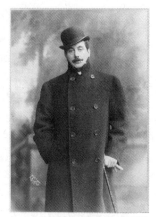

Giacomo Puccini, 1908.

In 1919, Surrealist artist Marcel Duchamp sketched a mustache (and goatee) on a postcard of the Mona Lisa with the letters L.H.O.O.Q. on the bottom. It is speculated that pronouncing each letter in French produces a slangish homophone for *"elle a chaud au cul"* (translation: "she has a hot ass"). Was he the inspiration for countless other mo-spraying graffiti artists in the early twenty-first century?

THE SPORTY MO

Male athletes help us to construct notions of masculinity, male bonding, and physical prowess. We idealize them, imitate them, and follow their every move. We even grow mo's and beards along with them when they are participating in the post-season playoffs as a brotherly sign of team loyalty and devotion. See if you agree with our choices for Number One Mustache Guy in baseball, American football, and hockey.

TEN GREATEST MUSTACHES IN BASEBALL HISTORY

Men in baseball were the first to sport the stache, even though team owners didn't always approve. One exception was Charlie Finley, the owner of the Oakland Athletics in the 1970s, who held a stache-growing contest among his players. When the A's faced the baby-faced Cincinnati Reds in the 1972 World Series, media outlets called it "the hairs versus the squares."

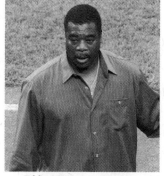

Eddie Murray at a ceremony at Camden Yards in 2007. Photo, Keith Allison.

10. Eddie "Steady Eddie" Murray (Baltimore Orioles)

9. Mike Schmidt (Philadelphia Phillies)

8. James "Catfish" Hunter (Oakland Athletics; New York Yankees)

7. James Francis "Pud" Galvin (St. Louis Browns)

6. Randy Johnson (Atlanta Braves)

5. Dave Stieb (Toronto Blue Jays)

4. Al Hrabosky (St. Louis Cardinals)

3. Richard "Goose" Gossage (New York Yankees; San Diego Padres)

2. Keith Hernandez (New York Mets)

1. Roland "Rollie" Fingers (Oakland Athletics; Milwaukee Brewers)

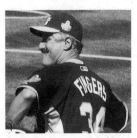

Rollie Fingers at the 2008 Allstars and Legends game at Yankee Stadium.

The stache was popular in the early days of baseball but fell into disfavor for a time in 1900. This was apocryphally blamed on Giants outfielder Jim O'Rourke, for losing a ball because his stache supposedly got in the way!

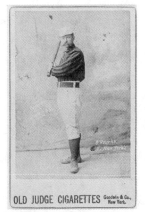

OLD JUDGE CIGARETTES Goodwin & Co., New York.

Jim O'Rourke, left fielder, 1888.

TEN GREATEST MUSTACHES IN US FOOTBALL HISTORY

The mustache has graced the faces of many American football greats. Bet you have no problem picturing the face of our number-one choice:

10. Harry Carson (New York Giants)

9. Marvin Harrison (Indianapolis Colts)

8. Dave Wannstedt
   (Buffalo Bills)

7. Nick Lowery
   (Kansas City Chiefs)

6. Walter Payton
   (Chicago Bears)

5. Ben Davidson
   (Oakland Raiders)

4. Cliff Harris
   (Dallas Cowboys)

3. Conrad Dobler
   (St. Louis Cardinals)

2. Mike Ditka (Chicago Bears, and others, player and coach)

1. Joe Namath (New York Jets)

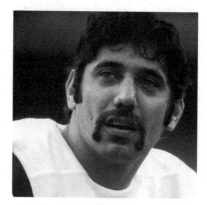

Joe Namath, quarterback for the NY Jets 1965–1976.

Joe Namath shaved off his Fu Manchu stache on December 11, 1968. He used a heavily advertised Schick razor and was paid $10,000, or about $10 per hair!

"It's magic. You just have to pet it, take care of it. You trim the mustache so it doesn't hang on your lip. Then you just make sure you stroke it and keep it nice."
—Brett Keisel (Pittsburgh Steelers)

TEN GREATEST MUSTACHES IN HOCKEY HISTORY

Players in the National Hockey League are well-known for its play-off beards (i.e., players in the National Hockey League stop shaving so as not to lose their mo-jo during the annual lead-up to the Stanley Cup). In April 2011, Brian Boyle of the New York Rangers caused a sensation when he grew a playoff stache, as his beard wasn't full enough. Over the years, a few other brave souls (many of them Canadian) have eschewed chin hair but celebrated their furry lips.

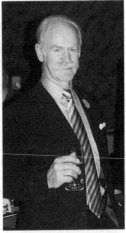

10. Paul MacLean (Winnipeg Jets)
9. Dennis Maruk (Washington Capitals)
8. Garth Boesch (Toronto Maple Leafs)
7. Harold Snepsts (Vancouver Canucks)
6. George Parros (Anaheim Ducks)
5. Rod Langway (Washington Capitals)
4. Grant Fuhr (Edmonton Oilers)
3. Pat Burns (coach, Montreal Canadiens, Toronto Maple Leafs, and others)
2. Wendel Clark (Toronto Maple Leafs)
1. Lanny McDonald (Toronto Maple Leafs)

Lanny McDonald at Canada's Sports Hall of Fame Induction Dinner, November 10, 2010, Calgary, Alberta.

OTHER SPORTY STACHES:

Basketball:
Kareem Abdul-Jabbar
Charles Barkley
Brad Davis
Joe Dumars
A.C. Green
Adam Morrison

Boxing:
George Foreman
Don King (promoter)
Ken Norton
Sugar Ray Robinson

Car Racing:
Dale Earnhardt, Sr.
Jeff Gordon
Richard Lee Petty

Golf:
John Ball, Jr.
Andres Gonzales
Montford Johnson Wagner

Soccer/football
Phillippe Albert
George Best
Humberto Coelho
Gary Neville
Graeme Souness
Rudi Voeller

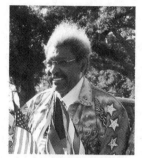

American boxing promotor Don King during a tour of Hurlburt Field, Florida.

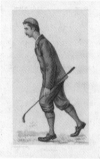

Caricature of Mr. John Ball Jr. by Liborio Prosperi, 1892.

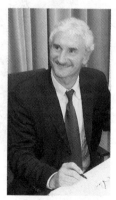

Rudi Voeller. Photo, Tobias Koch, 2002.

Swimming:
John Naber
Michael Phelps
Mark Spitz

**"When I went to the Olympics, I had every intention of shaving the mustache off, but I realized I was getting so many comments about it—and everybody was talking about it—that I decided to keep it."
—Mark Spitz**

Wrestling:
Hulk Hogan (Terry Gene Bollea)
The Iron Sheik (Hossein Khosrow Ali Vaziri)
Ravishing Rick Rude (Richard Erwin Rood)

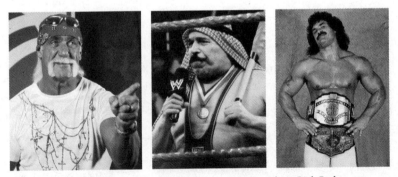

Hulk Hogan, 2006, The Iron Shiek at WWE Raw, 2008, Ravishing Rick Rude.

THE POMO MO

The 1990s paved the way for a facial-hair explosion not seen since Victorian times. Kurt Cobain and other grunge rock types grew wisps and goatees, of which variants were then swiftly adopted by all ethnicities and ages in the global community. In previous eras, men took their fashion cues from clergymen, royalty, and politicians, but now rock stars, actors, athletes, and the latest looks on the fashion runway were the go-to source for manly style, including facial hair. As the goatee became ubiquitous (worn even by fathers and grandfathers), twentysomethings then began to explore every permutation and combination of sideburns, mustaches, beards, and chin dots imaginable—and the possibilities were endless. But there was another key difference—postmodern facial hair was clearly being worn ironically, with a wink of the eye. New and playful trends, such as playoff beards, strike beards, layoff beards, break-up beards, and f-u beards, have since emerged and mustache charity movements have started sweeping the globe (see Appendix, p.142).

Some believe that this latest wave of facial hairiness is a post-feminist expression, that is, men are growing something on their faces that (most) women could not, for facial hair is indubitably testosterone-driven. Nonetheless, it can now be said that facial hair has become something of the norm for men worldwide, particularly young, urban ones. (If you don't believe me, count the furry faces on the streets in your town, in other cities when you travel and in sports, fashion, and athletic magazines.) Increasingly, professional men, like their Victorian forefathers, are proud mo-growers too. College kids are braiding their facial hair and growing Fu Manchus or sprouting full cathedral beards. Hipsters sport straggly beards and mustaches. The clean-shaven metro-sexual is no longer dominant (thank God!) although they gave men the confidence to buy and use lavish grooming products.

<hr/>

The Mo as Wife Magnet: A 2001 study by Nigel Barber published in the *Journal of Nonverbal Behavior* demonstrated that the mustache has been consistently associated with enhancing marriage prospects "by increasing physical attractiveness and perception of social status." Take note: beards and sideburns do not enjoy as strong an association, proving that potential mates of all genders have long warmed up to the mustache's charms.

When you think of it, though, it was really only a matter of time until the mustache became stylish again. As we have seen, the mo has been demeaned and belittled on a cyclical basis throughout history as the domain of fops, foreigners, and fiends (not to mention porn stars, gay clones, and overly independent free-thinkers). But postmodern men, confident in their own masculinity, are now able to grow, twirl, and twiddle their fine staches without fear of reproach; they're okay with enduring multiple interpretations (even blatantly wrong ones) of what their mo's must really "mean."

Charity movements like Movember allow men of all ages to grow their mustaches for good causes for a finite period of time but many use them as an excuse to start a mo and then keep it long after the fundraising has ended. Postmodern men seem willing to forget or deconstruct all the historical baggage that comes with the mo and embrace the sexy, comical, ambiguous, and macho all at once.

"Like two erect sentries, my mustache defends the entrance to my real self." —Salvador Dali

As always, the shaving industry, of course, would like to see us all clean-shaven. But as a testament to the persistence and durability of the latest facial-hair craze, most companies have released products with features that allow you to shape, trim, or decide (within a millimeter) the length of your chosen stache style. (And, if you're a purist, you do need to close-shave the rest of your face.) And in Hollywood, a rash of A-list actors (see list following) are becoming increasingly attached to the mustaches they grow for specific roles.

Clearly, a handsome face can be made even more handsome with a mustache. The mustache may be a perfect, postmodern symbol of masculinity: playful, ironic, virile, independent, and, above all, sociable. Men of the mustache make up a new fraternity, one of the few, non-militaristic options for male bonding across age, sexual orientation, and ethnicity. Long-term mustache wearers, like firemen, African-American men, and men from stache-friendly countries like India or Turkey rarely say, "I told you so," or "What kept you?" Instead, they are welcoming their newly enlightened mo-bros with open arms!

CONTEMPORARY ACTOR STACHES

- Orlando Bloom
- Josh Brolin
- Pierce Brosnan
- George Clooney
- Billy Crudup
- Daniel Day-Lewis
- Robert Downey, Jr.
- Zac Efron
- Michael Fassbender
- James Franco
- Ryan Gosling
- Ashton Kutcher
- Jude Law
- Viggo Mortensen
- Eddie Murphy
- Clive Owen
- Sean Penn
- Brad Pitt
- Jason Schwartzman
- Will Smith

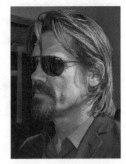

Josh Brolin at the 2010 Toronto International Film Festival. Photo, gdcgraphics.

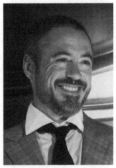

Robert Downey Jr. promoting the film *Iron Man* in Mexico City, 2008. Photo, Edgar Meritano.

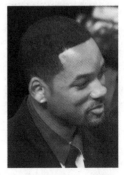

Will Smith at Nobel Peace Prize, 2009. Photo, Harry Wad.

Most workplaces, with the possible exceptions of those in government and banking, have removed obstacles from employees wishing to wear the mustache. Pockets of discrimination, however, still exist; for example, you are unlikely to be chosen for jury duty if you have a mustache, and if you are a clergyman, your congregation may never trust you. Postmodern men, however, are seldom wed to a single furry expression. Facial hair is a highly individualistic art form, and many men continue to change their look to mark transitions in their working and personal lives. Teenaged boys beam with pride at the external expression of their newly flowing testosterone, even while their parents beg them to shave. Twentysomethings might wear the mustache to look older and (they hope) "hotter." Men in their thirties may choose to wear a mo to look younger, or to counteract age-related changes in their faces. As they get older, some men will even expressly mimic cultural heroes like Mark Twain or Salvador Dali. Guys in their forties and beyond are also known to dye their staches if they go grey or whiten.

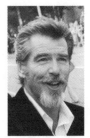

Pierce Brosnan, 2005. Photo, Sheksays.

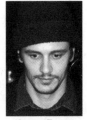

James Franco, 2011. Photo, Tony Shek.

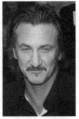

Sean Penn, 2006. Photo, Attit Patel.

Only the man who grows a mustache knows why he has done so. Even then, his reasons may not be fully conscious or informed by historical knowledge, though we used to be able to read a man's allegiances, politics, and class by the shape and size of his stache. In our increasingly egalitarian, multicultural, media-mad society, anything goes. A man may actually be saying or projecting more

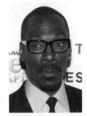

Eddie Murphy, 2010. Photo, David Shankbone

than one thing with his mustache, which makes it a power-ful performance of his notions of masculinity and his unique place in the world.

However, if this new wave of mustaches becomes too ubiq-uitous, it may again vanish. But fear not. The stache will always return with a vengeance as the final, furry frontier. After all, no other male statement is as ambiguous, playful, mysterious, masculine, or misunderstood. And any one of those is reason enough to start growing your own mo!

A GALLERY OF STACHE STYLES

Some (spite their teeth) like thatch'd eaves downward grows

And some grow upward in despite their nose;

Some their moustaches of such length do keep,

That very well they may a manger sweep,

Which in beer, ale, or wine they drinking plunge,

And suck the liquor up as 'twere a sponge.

But 'tis sloven's beastly pride, I think,

To wash his beard where other men must drink.

And some, (because they will not rob the cup)

Their upper chops like pot hooks are turned up.

The barbers thus (like tailors) still must be

Acquainted with each cut's variety.

"Superbiae Flagellum, Or, The Whip of Pride"
—John Taylor, 1621

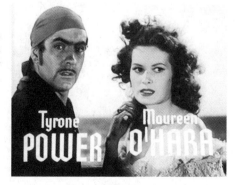

Tyrone Power and Maureen O'Hara in a screenshot from the trailer for the film *The Black Swan*, 1942.

AN A–Z OF MUSTACHE STYLES THROUGH THE AGES

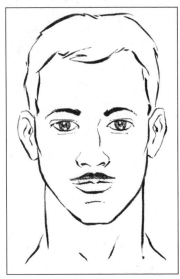

ADOLPHE MENJOU

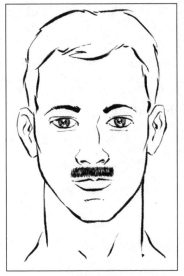

BOX CAR

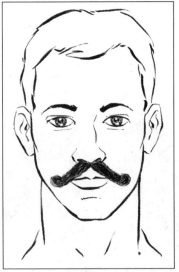

BULLET HEADS

BUTTONS

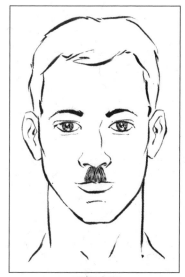

CHAPLIN
(also known as the Tramp or Toothbrush)

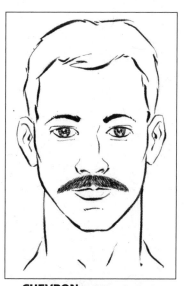

CHEVRON (a fuller take on the Military; also known as the Magnum)

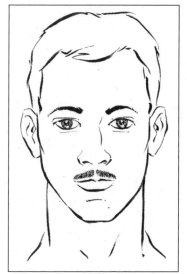

CLARK GABLE
(also known as the Thin Lizzy)

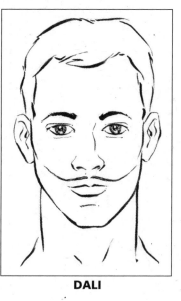

DALI

A Gallery of Stache Styles **127**

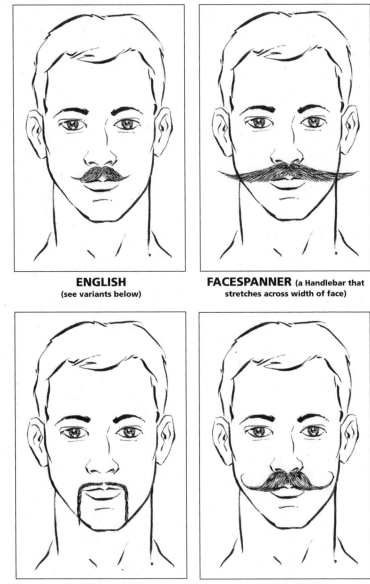

ENGLISH
(see variants below)

FACESPANNER (a Handlebar that
stretches across width of face)

FU MANCHU
(also known as Fu Tang)

HANDLEBAR
(also known as the Howie or Wild West)

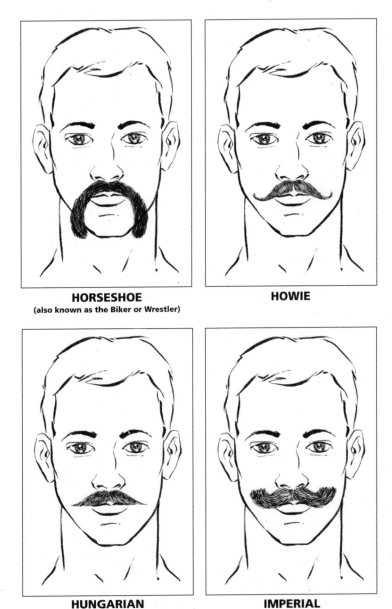

HORSESHOE
(also known as the Biker or Wrestler)

HOWIE

HUNGARIAN

IMPERIAL

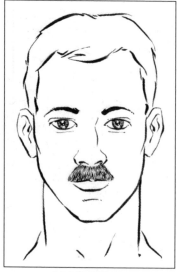

LAMPSHADE

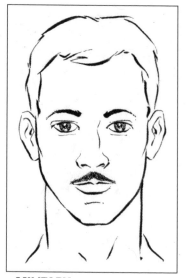

MILITARY (also known as the Cop
Stache, or the Battle; see English variants)

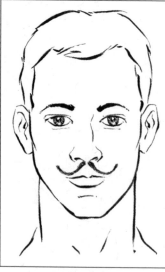

MISTLETOE

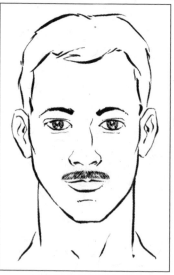

PAINTER'S BRUSH

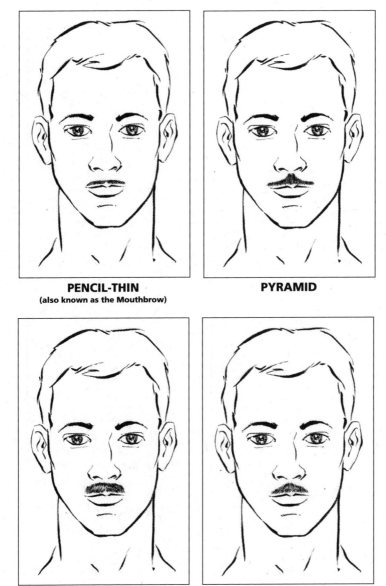

PENCIL-THIN
(also known as the Mouthbrow)

PYRAMID

REGENT

SHERMANIC

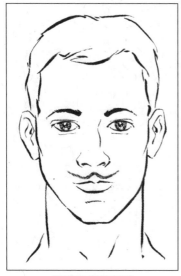

STRIP-TEASER

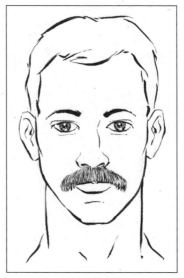

WALRUS

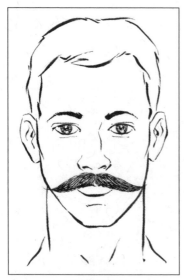

ZAPATA

"I added a small moustache, which I reasoned would add age without hiding my expression." —Charlie Chaplin, *My Autobiography*

ENGLISH MUSTACHE VARIANTS

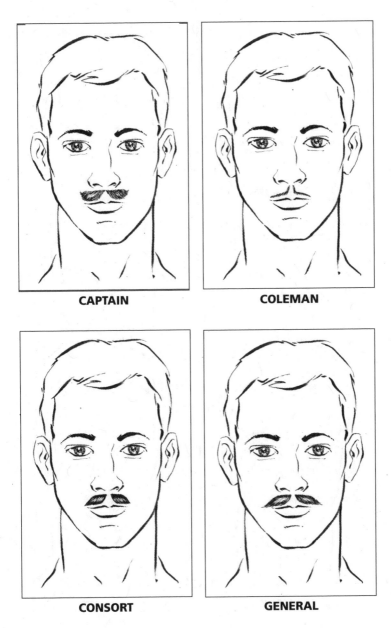

CAPTAIN

COLEMAN

CONSORT

GENERAL

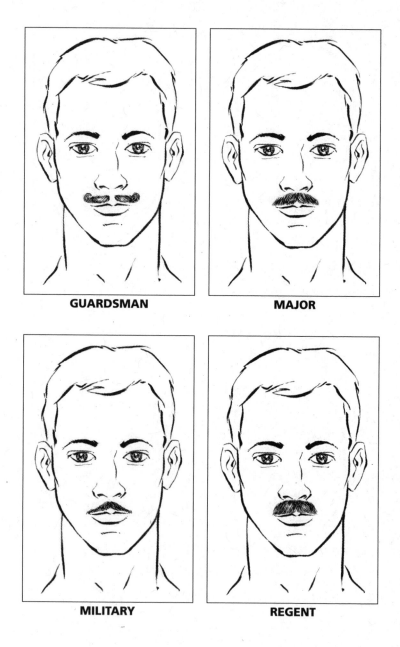

GUARDSMAN

MAJOR

MILITARY

REGENT

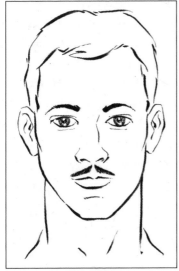

SHADOW

"A man wears a mustache because there's something he wants to conceal... a spiritual defect."
—Ayn Rand

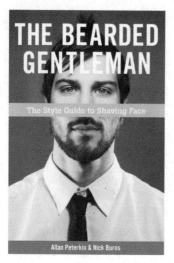

For mo' hands-on groovy/ styling tips for your stache, go to *The Bearded Gentleman: The Style Guide to Shaving Face* **by Peterkin & Burns, 2010. beardedgentleman.com**

MO' MO: AN APPENDIX OF ADDITIONAL INFORMATION

Certain chaps never gave up on their staches, even when the going got tough. These five organizations deserve credit for paving the way for the millennial mustache. Check out their websites for spectacular mo trivia and brotherhood.

1. THE HANDLEBAR CLUB (HANDLEBARCLUB.CO.UK)

The Handlebar Club was founded in April 1947 in the dressing room of comedian Jimmy Edwards at the Windmill Theatre in London. The ten founding members were, according to club archives, "outnumbered by chorus girls!"

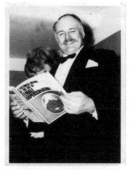

Jimmy Edwards. Photo, Chris Shaw.

Since its inception, the Handlebar Club has brought together mustache wearers in a social context to support worthy charities and causes, particularly those devoted to children and veterans. Beard-wearers, however, are strictly forbidden.

By the 1960s, membership peaked at about 200, with informal meetings taking place on the first Friday of each month. These meetings traditionally occured at the Pathfinder Club, but have since moved to the Windsor Castle pub in Crawford Place, London.

Founder Edwards withdrew from active membership in 1968, the club's twenty-first anniversary. As the club grew, branches developed to accommodate members who could not travel to the monthly meetings. As of 2011, three such branches—known to members as nests—continue to operate, in the East Midlands (UK), Sweden, and Norway. These nests conduct their own activities whilst keeping in close contact with the main club in London.

A period of dwindling membership was followed by a resurgence in the 1980s, ushering in a more formal administrative structure and a regular newsletter which keeps members abreast of events. In the 1980s, the Handlebar Club also began networking with European mustache clubs, and through the next decades, figured prominently at international mustache competitions, hosting the 2007 World Beard and Moustache Championships.

Women are now admitted to monthly meetings, and there has been a transition from more "active" sports to the more moderate pastime of darts. The club hosts other local social clubs at charity challenges and raffles. Today, the Handlebar Club has 100 members.

‎◆ ● ◆‎

The Barbershop Harmony Society (*barbershop.org*), founded in 1938, has 30,000 members. It relocated its headquarters from Wisconsin to Nashville in 2007. Straw hats, colorful vests, a bowtie, and big ol' staches make up the standard uniform. Another international group of stache-wearing singers is the Barbershop Quartet Preservation Association (*bqpa.com*).

2. AMERICAN MUSTACHE INSTITUTE
(AMERICANMUSTACHEINSTITUTE.ORG)

Founded in 1965, the American Mustache Institute is the world's leading facial hair advocacy organization, protecting the rights of, and fighting discrimination against, mustached Americans. According to its website, the AMI is "broadly considered the bravest organization in the history of mankind (behind only the US military and the post-Jim Henson Muppets), the Institute serves as the ACLU of the downtrodden mustached American people. Its headquarters are in the city of St. Louis, home to the world's largest mustache—the Gateway Arch."

3. WORLD BEARD AND MOUSTACHE CHAMPIONSHIPS
(WORLDBEARDCHAMPIONSHIPS.COM)

According to its website, the origins of the World Beard and Moustache Championships is hotly disputed. The Italian delegation claims that the first championships took place in Northern Italy in the early 1970s, but the event as it is known today is allegedly traceable to a 1990 event hosted by the First Höfener Beard Club, at Höfen an der Enz, Germany, a small village near the Black Forest. In 1995, the same club hosted the second World Beard and Moustache Championships in the nearby city of Pforzheim.

Since 1995, the championships have been held every two years, migrating across Europe through Germany, Norway, Sweden, and back to Germany in 2001, when the Swabian Beard and Moustache Club celebrated its tenth anniversary by hosting the championships in Schömberg.

In 2003, the championships were held outside Europe for

the first time, at Carson City, Nevada. Approximately eighty-five Europeans took part, with a strong showing from the German delegates, who won thirty-six of the fifty-seven trophies awarded. It is customary for each competition to feature beards sculpted and styled in homage to architectural wonders of the host city; among the stand-outs were the Brandenburg Gate (2005), the Golden Gate Bridge (2003), and London's Tower Bridge (2007).

Germany continued its domination through 2005 and 2007, at which point Beard Team USA showcased some strong whiskers. By 2009, the USA emerged as the "world's new facial hair super-power," winning in several categories at the Championships in Anchorage, Alaska. Beard Team USA ("For Mustaches Too") has held annual National Beard and Mustache Championships in the US and now has over 100 local chapters. In North America, we owe much to them for paving the way for furry liberation and celebration!

4. MOVEMBER (MOVEMBER.COM)

Movember (a portmanteau of "mo" for mustache and "November") is an annual, month-long fundraising event for prostate cancer research in which participants around the world grow and wear mustaches during the month of November. The campaign helps to encourage men to visit the doctor, increase their awareness of family medical histories, and adopt healthier lifestyles, resulting in increased early cancer detection, diagnosis and effective treatments, and ultimately a reduction in the number of preventable deaths. Participants, colloquially known as "mo bros," effectively become advocates for men's health, prompting private and public conversation around this often ignored issue.

Founded in Adelaide, Australia, in 1999, Movember originally boasted eighty members and aimed to raise funds for the Royal Society for the Prevention of Cruelty to Animals, under the slogan, "Growing whiskers for whiskers." In 2004, the group officially became the Movember Foundation, with charitable status and a focus on issues of men's health. By 2007, local chapters had formed in New Zealand, Ireland, Canada, the Czech Republic, Denmark, Spain, the United Kingdom, Israel, South Africa, Taiwan, and the United States. The year 2010 saw the Movember Foundation merge with TacheBack, a charitable group founded in the UK with a commitment to raising awareness about prostate and testicular cancers. As of 2011, Canadians were the largest contributors to Movember charities of any nation.

5. THE GLORIUS MUSTACHE CHALLENGE (GLORIUSMUSTACHE.COM)

A documentary conceived, produced, and directed by Jay Della Valle, *The Glorius Mustache Challenge* is self-defined as "a social engineering experiment designed to rescue the sexy mustache from the pop culture graveyard."

In 2004, Della Valle issued a challenge to American men under the age of thirty, printed on handbills and distributed in the streets: grow a mustache for one month, beginning with a clean-shaven face. The resulting film explores the social anxieties, insecurities, and excitement of the participants, and features a fun animated history of the mustache.

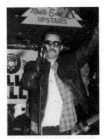

Jay Della Valle playing at The Middle East (Cambridge, MA), 2009.

FUNDRAISERS/ CHARITABLE ORGANIZATIONS

Fund-a-Stache: *fundastache.org* (see site for selected charities, guidelines, and dates)

Movember/TacheBack: *movember.com* (see site for local chapters, worldwide)

Mustaches for Kids: *mustachesforkids.org* (see site for local chapters across North America)

INTERNATIONAL CLUBS

World Beard and Moustache Championships: *worldbeardchampionships.com*

Belgium:
Snorrenclub Anterwerpen: *snorrenclubantwerpen.be*

Canada:
Beard Team Canada: *beardteamcanada.com*

France:
Association les Moustachus d'Alsace: *moustachusalsace.free.fr*

Germany:
Association of German Beard Clubs (Hoefener Bart-und Schnorresclub): *bartclub.de*

Italy:
Baffomania: *baffomania.it*

Netherlands:
Snorrenclub Flevoland: *snorrenclubflevoland.nl*

Norway:
Den Norske Mustach-Club av-91: *dnm91.com*

Sweden:

Svenska Mustaschklubben: *mustascher.se*

Switzerland:

Schnauz-und Bartclub Rheintal: *bart.li/startseitescbr.htm*

United Kingdom:

The Handlebar Club: *handlebarclub.co.uk*

United States:

American Mustache Institute: *americanmustacheinstitute.org*

Beard Team USA: *beardteamusa.org* (also includes links to almost fifty local and national stache and beard clubs)

The Glorius Mustache Challenge: *gloriusmustache.com*

Order of the Hirsute: *orderofthehirsute.com*

Whisker Club: *whiskerclub.org*

SPORTS MUSTACHE SITES

A Stash of Sports Staches (ABC News): *abcnews.go.com/Sports/popup?id=5357240*

Joe Pelletier's Greatest Hockey Legends: *greatesthockeylegends.com/2008/09/top-ten-mustaches-in-hockey-history.html*

Bleacher Report: *bleacherreport.com/articles/579591-carl-pavano-and-the-10-greatest-mustaches-in-baseball-history*

MISCELLANEOUS SITES

The Art of Manliness: *artofmanliness.com*

Beard Team USA: *beardteamusa.org*

Beardhead: *beardhead.com* (click on "staches")

Below the Nose: *belowthenose.blogspot.com*

Gentleman's Emporium: *gentlemansemporium.com* (click on "Stage Mustaches")

Moustache Me: *moustacheme.com*

Moustache Mojo: *moustachemojo.com*

Mustaches of the Nineteenth Century: *mustachesofthenineteenthcentury.blogspot.com*

REFERENCES

BOOKS:

Andrews, William. *At the Sign of the Barber's Pole: Studies in Hirsute History*. Yorkshire: JR Tutin, 1904.

Biddle-Perry, Geraldine and Sarah Cheang. *Hair: Styling, Culture and Fashion*. New York: Berg, 2008.

Charles, Ann and DeAnfrasio, Roger. *The History of Hair: An Illustrated Review of Hair Fashions For Men throughout the Ages*. New York: Bonanza Books, 1970.

Chattman, Jon and Rich Tarantino, et al. *Sweet Stache: 50 Badass Mustaches and the Faces Who Sport Them*. Avon, MA: Adams Media, 2009.

Corson, Richard. *Fashions in Hair: The First Five Thousand Years*. London: Peter Owen Limited, 2000.

Dali, Salvador and Phillipe Halsman. *Dali's Mustache*. Paris: Flammarion, 1954.

Dunkling, Leslie and John Foley. *Guinness Book of Beards and Moustaches*. London: Guinness Publishing, 1990.

Dutton, Paul Edward. *Charlemagne's Mustache: And Other Cultural Clusters of a Dark Age*. New York: Palgrave MacMillan, 2008.

Editors of Esquire Magazine. *Esquire: The Handbook of Style: A Man's Guide to Looking Good*. New York: Hearst Books, 2009.

Edwards, Lucien. *The Moustache Grower's Guide.* Chronicle Books, 2011.

Knowles, Elizabeth, ed. *The Oxford Dictionary of Quotations.* New York: Oxford University Press, 2009.

Morris, Desmond. *The Naked Man: A Study of the Male Body.* New York: Vintage Books, 2009.

Peterkin, Allan. *One Thousand Beards: A Cultural History of Facial Hair.* Vancouver: Arsenal Pulp Press, 2001.

Peterkin, Allan and Burns, Nick. *The Bearded Gentleman: The Style Guide To Shaving Face.* Vancouver: Arsenal Pulp Press, 2010.

Reynolds, Reginald. *Beards.* Indiana: Harcourt Brace Jovanovich, 1976.

Sherrow, Victoria. *Encyclopedia of Hair: A Cultural History.* London: Greenwood Press, 2006.

Taylor, Terry. *Stache: Frivolous Facts & Fancies About That Space Between the Nose and Lip.* New York: Lark Crafts, 2010.

VIDEOS:

The Glorius Mustache Challenge. DVD. Directed by Jay Della Valle.[n.l.]: Reel Eyez Films, 2007.

PERIODICAL ARTICLES:

Barber, Nigel. "Mustache Fashion Covaries with a Good Marriage Market for Women." *Journal of Nonverbal Behavior* 25, no. 4 (Winter 2001).

Brendon, Piers. "How the Moustache Won an Empire." *Daily Mail* (October 11, 2007). http://www.dailymail.co.uk/news/article-486942/How-moustache-won-empire.html.

Burns, Nick. "One Hairy Lip: A Mix of Messages." *The New York Times* (November 2, 2006): E3.

Dixson, Barnaby and Paul L. Vasey. "Beards Augment Perceptions of Men's Age, Social Status, and Aggressiveness, but Not Attractiveness." *Behavioral Ecology* (January 13, 2012). doi:10.1093/beheco/arr214.

Efron, Edith. "Saga of the Mustache: To Shave or Not To Shave?" *The New York Times* (August 20, 1944): SM20.

Esquire Staff. "Facial Fur Tache Back." *Esquire* (May 2009): 143.

Oldstone-Moore, Christopher. "Mustaches and Masculine Codes in Early Twentieth-Century America." *Journal of Social History* 45, no. 1 (Fall 2011): 47–60.

Rimer, Sarah. "The Fireman's Mustache: Badge of the Brotherhood." *The New York Times* (June 21, 1986). http://www.nytimes.com/1986/06/21/nyregion/the-fireman-s-mustache-badge-of-the-brotherhood.html.

Shelton, Karen Marie. "Men's Facial Hair: Mustaches Designs." *Hair-Boutique.com* (December 15, 2003). http://www.hairboutique.com/tips/articles.php?f=tip3907.html.

Vierra, Dan. "Mustaches Are Growing in Popularity." *Arizona Daily Star*, (December 11, 2006). http://azstarnet.com/allheadlines/159599.

Walton, Susan. "From Squalid Impropriety to Manly Respectability: The Revival of Beards, Moustaches and Martial Values in the 1850s in England." *Nineteenth-Century Contexts* 30, no. 3 (September 2008): 229–45.

WEB REFERENCES
(IN ADDITION TO THOSE MENTIONED ABOVE):

A Lust for Lists: Ten Political Moustaches: *a-lust-for-lists.blogspot.com/2011/04/ten-political-moustaches.html*

Art History Club: Moustache in Art History: *arthistoryclub.com/art_history/Moustache*

The Bearded Gentleman: *www.beardedgentleman.com*

The Dandy: The Meaning of the Moustache: *thedandy.org/themeaningofthemoustache*

Encyclopaedia Britannica: Mustache: *britannica.com/EBchecked/topic/399541/mustache*

IBN Live: Top Ten Moustache-dense Nations for Movember: *ibnlive.in.com/news/travel-picks-top-10-moustachedense-nations-for-movember/104682-26.html*

Öğret, Özgür. "Facial Hair in Turkish Politics: A Tale of Mustaches and Men." *Hurriet Daily News*, (August 6, 2010). *hurriyetdailynews.com/default.aspx?pageid=438&n=facial-hair-in-turkish-politics-a-tale-of-moustaches-and-men-2010-08-06*

Stachist: Mustache History: *stachist.com/category/mustache-history/*

Ultimate Classic Rock: Top Ten Rock Mustaches: *ultimate-classicrock.com/rock-mustaches/*

US Air Force Grooming Standards: *usmilitary.about.com/cs/airforce/a/afgrooming.html*

Wikipedia.org: Facial Hair in the Military: *en.wikipedia.org/wiki/Facial_hair_in_the_military*

Wikipedia.org: Notable Moustaches: *en.wikipedia.org/wiki/Moustache*

Wikipedia.org: Moustache cups: *en.wikipedia.org/wiki/Moustache_cup*

INDEX

NOTE: Page numbers in *italics* indicate photographs or illustrations. Page numbers in **bold** denote stache style illustrations.

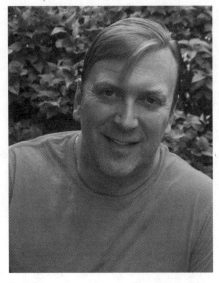

ALLAN PETERKIN is a psychiatrist living in Toronto and the author of the bestselling *One Thousand Beards: A Cultural History of Facial Hair* as well as six other books on cultural history and medicine; he is also co-author (with Nick Burns) of *The Bearded Gentleman: The Style Guide to Shaving Face.* His comments on facial hair have been published in *Esquire, Men's Health,* the *Wall Street Journal,* the *Financial Times,* the *New Yorker,* the *New York Times, Sports Illustrated,* and *US,* as well as in the film documentary *Mansome.*